ASTHMA? NO PROBLEM!

YOUR GUIDE TO A BREATHTAKING LIFE

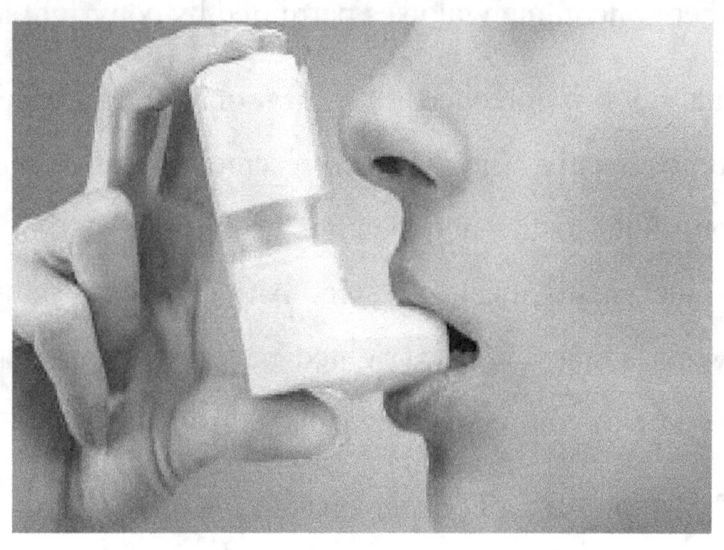

BY: DR. JADEN CLINTON

TABLE OF CONTENT

INTRODUCTION

Asthma might seem like an insurmountable challenge, but it doesn't have to be. With the right knowledge and proactive steps, you can transform your experience with asthma and embrace a life full of vitality and freedom. This book is your roadmap to achieving just that—a breathtaking life where asthma is no longer a hindrance but a manageable aspect of your daily routine.

Imagine waking up every morning without the fear of an impending asthma attack. Picture yourself engaging in your favorite activities, whether it's hiking up a scenic trail, playing with your kids in the park, or simply enjoying a leisurely stroll through your neighborhood. This reality is entirely possible, and this book will show you how to get there.

Asthma is more than just a respiratory condition; it's a call to understand your body better, to recognize the triggers, and to develop strategies that keep you in control. In these pages, you'll uncover the secrets to effective asthma management and prevention, empowering you to take charge of your health and well-being.

You'll explore the latest research, practical tips, and inspiring stories of individuals who have conquered their asthma challenges. From dietary changes and exercise routines to medication management and stress reduction techniques, every chapter is designed to arm you with tools and insights that make living with asthma not only manageable but truly enjoyable.

We'll travel through the science of asthma, shedding light on what happens in your body during an asthma attack and how you can prevent it. You'll learn about the environmental and lifestyle factors that play a significant role in asthma management, and how simple adjustments can make a world of difference.

Additionally, this guide will offer you a comprehensive plan tailored to your unique needs. Whether you're newly diagnosed or have been living with asthma for years, you'll find strategies to enhance your quality of life. From building a support network to creating an asthma-friendly home, every aspect of your life will be considered to ensure you can breathe easier and live better.

Asthma? No problem! Together, we will unlock the potential for a healthier, happier, and more fulfilling life. Prepare to embark on a transformative journey where asthma becomes just a small part of your extraordinary life story.

CHAPTER ONE

DEMYSTIFYING ASTHMA

1.1 WHAT IS ASTHMA AND HOW DOES IT WORK?

Asthma is a chronic respiratory condition that affects millions of people worldwide. It's characterized by inflammation and narrowing of the airways, which makes breathing difficult. To truly understand asthma, it's important to look at the mechanics of the condition, the different types of asthma, and how they manifest in everyday life.

The Mechanics of Asthma

At its core, asthma is a condition that impacts the bronchial tubes, the airways that carry air in and out of your lungs. In a person with asthma, these airways are often inflamed and can become even more swollen and constricted in response to various triggers. This narrowing of the airways reduces the flow of air and causes the classic symptoms of asthma: wheezing, shortness of breath, chest tightness, and coughing.

When the bronchial tubes are exposed to an asthma trigger—such as allergens, cold air, or physical activity—they react by tightening the surrounding muscles, swelling, and producing excess mucus. This three-pronged attack significantly restricts airflow and makes breathing a strenuous task.

To visualize this, think of trying to breathe through a straw while pinching it tighter and tighter. The effort required to pull air through the narrowed tube is much greater, leading to fatigue and discomfort.

Different Types of Asthma and Their Characteristics

Asthma isn't a one-size-fits-all condition; it presents itself in various forms, each with its unique characteristics. Understanding the type of asthma you or a loved one has can help tailor a more effective management plan.

1. Allergic Asthma: This is the most common type and is triggered by allergens such as pollen, pet dander, dust mites, and mold. People with allergic asthma often have other allergic conditions like eczema or hay fever.

2. Non-Allergic Asthma: This type is triggered by factors not related to allergies, such as stress, exercise, cold air, or respiratory infections. Non-allergic asthma tends to be more prevalent in adults.

3. Exercise-Induced Bronchoconstriction (EIB): Often referred to as exercise-induced asthma, EIB is characterized by airway constriction that occurs during or after physical exertion. Symptoms typically start a few minutes into exercise and can last for up to an hour.

4. Occupational Asthma: This type is caused by workplace irritants such as chemicals, dust, or gases. Symptoms often improve when away from the work environment.

5. Nocturnal Asthma: Asthma symptoms that worsen at night are referred to as nocturnal asthma. This can disrupt sleep and significantly impact quality of life. Triggers

might include allergens, cooling of the airways, or reclining position.

6. Cough-Variant Asthma: Unlike typical asthma, where wheezing is a primary symptom, cough-variant asthma is characterized mainly by a persistent, dry cough. This type of asthma can be harder to diagnose.

Understanding which type of asthma, you have is crucial because it influences both the triggers to avoid and the treatments that will be most effective.

Recognizing Asthma Symptoms and Triggers

Asthma symptoms can vary widely in frequency and severity. Some people experience mild symptoms occasionally, while others may have severe, daily symptoms. The common symptoms include:

- Wheezing: A high-pitched whistling sound made while breathing, particularly when exhaling.
- Shortness of Breath: Feeling like you can't get enough air, which can be especially pronounced during physical activity or at night.

- Chest Tightness: A sensation of pressure or squeezing in the chest.
- Coughing: Often worse at night or early morning, and can be persistent.

Identifying your asthma triggers is a key part of managing the condition. Triggers can vary from person to person, but common ones include:

Allergens: Pollen, dust mites, pet dander, and mold.

1. Irritants: Tobacco smoke, pollution, strong odors, and chemical fumes.

2. Respiratory Infections: Colds, flu, and other infections can exacerbate asthma symptoms.

3. Physical Activity: Exercise, particularly in cold or dry air, can trigger symptoms.

4. Weather: Cold air, changes in weather, or even hot, humid conditions.

5. Emotions: Strong emotions and stress can lead to hyperventilation and trigger asthma symptoms.

Keeping a symptom diary can be a helpful tool in recognizing patterns and identifying specific triggers. Documenting when and where your symptoms occur, along with any potential triggers, can provide valuable insights for both you and your healthcare provider.

Understanding the nuances of asthma is the first step toward effective management. By recognizing the different types of asthma and their triggers, and being aware of your specific symptoms, you can work with your healthcare team to develop a personalized plan that helps you breathe easier and live a more fulfilling life.

Asthma might be a chronic condition, but with the right approach, it doesn't have to control your life.

1.2 Different types of asthma and their characteristics
Asthma is not a singular condition; it comes in various forms, each with its own unique triggers, symptoms, and management strategies. Understanding the different types of asthma can help you and your healthcare provider tailor an effective treatment plan that fits your specific needs.

Let's explore the primary types of asthma and what sets them apart.

Allergic Asthma

Allergic asthma, also known as atopic asthma, is the most common form of the condition. It is triggered by exposure to allergens—substances that cause an allergic reaction. These allergens can be found both indoors and outdoors and include pollen, pet dander, dust mites, and mold spores. People with allergic asthma often have a history of other allergic conditions such as eczema, hay fever, or allergic rhinitis.

Characteristics of Allergic Asthma:

Seasonal Variations: Symptoms may worsen during certain times of the year when specific allergens, like pollen, are more prevalent.

Associated Allergies: Patients often have other allergic symptoms such as sneezing, itchy eyes, and runny nose.

Response to Allergens: Symptoms typically occur soon after exposure to an allergen and can include wheezing, coughing, chest tightness, and shortness of breath.

Non-Allergic Asthma

Non-allergic asthma, or intrinsic asthma, is not related to allergens and can be triggered by factors such as stress, exercise, cold air, respiratory infections, or even certain medications. This type of asthma tends to develop later in life and can be more persistent and harder to control compared to allergic asthma.

Characteristics of Non-Allergic Asthma:

No Allergic Reaction: Symptoms are not triggered by allergens and patients often do not have other allergic conditions.

Environmental Triggers: Factors such as smoke, strong odors, weather changes, and respiratory infections are common triggers.

Consistent Symptoms: Unlike allergic asthma, which may have seasonal patterns, non-allergic asthma symptoms can occur year-round.

Exercise-Induced Bronchoconstriction (EIB)

Often referred to as exercise-induced asthma, EIB occurs when physical activity triggers airway constriction. Symptoms typically start a few minutes into exercise and can last for several minutes to an hour after stopping the activity. EIB is common in athletes and individuals who engage in vigorous physical activities, especially in cold or dry conditions.

Characteristics of EIB:

Timing of Symptoms: Symptoms begin during or shortly after exercise and include wheezing, shortness of breath, chest tightness, and coughing.

Cold or Dry Air: Exercising in cold or dry air can exacerbate symptoms.

Recovery Phase: Symptoms often improve with rest and the use of a bronchodilator before exercise can help prevent them.

Occupational Asthma

Occupational asthma is caused by inhaling fumes, gases, dust, or other potentially harmful substances while on the job. This type of asthma can develop in workers in a variety of industries, including manufacturing, agriculture, and healthcare. Symptoms often improve when the individual is away from the work environment, such as during weekends or vacations.

Characteristics of Occupational Asthma:

Workplace Exposure: Symptoms are directly related to exposure to specific substances at work.

Improvement Away from Work: Symptoms often lessen or disappear when not at the workplace.

Variety of Triggers: Common workplace triggers include chemicals, dust, mold, and animal proteins.

Nocturnal Asthma

Nocturnal asthma refers to asthma symptoms that worsen at night, disrupting sleep and significantly affecting quality of life. The exact cause of nocturnal asthma is not entirely understood, but it is believed to be related to the natural circadian rhythms, cooling of the airways during sleep, and reclining position.

Characteristics of Nocturnal Asthma:

Nighttime Symptoms: Increased coughing, wheezing, and shortness of breath during the night.

Impact on Sleep: Frequent nighttime awakenings and poor sleep quality.

Daytime Fatigue: Difficulty functioning during the day due to lack of restful sleep.

Cough-Variant Asthma

Cough-variant asthma is a form of asthma where the predominant symptom is a chronic, non-productive cough. This type of asthma can be particularly tricky to diagnose because it does not present with the typical wheezing or shortness of breath.

Characteristics of Cough-Variant Asthma:

Persistent Cough: A dry, hacking cough that lasts for more than eight weeks.

Absence of Wheezing: Unlike other forms of asthma, wheezing is not a common symptom.

Triggers Similar to Other Asthma Types: The cough can be triggered by the same factors that trigger other forms of asthma, such as allergens, exercise, and respiratory infections.

Understanding the type of asthma you have is crucial for effective management. It influences the triggers to avoid, the medications to use, and the lifestyle adjustments to make. Working closely with your healthcare provider to identify your asthma type can lead to a more tailored and effective treatment plan, ultimately improving your quality of life.

1.3 Recognizing asthma symptoms and triggers

Recognizing asthma symptoms and understanding what triggers them is fundamental to managing the condition effectively. Asthma symptoms can vary widely from person to person and even within the same individual over time. By being aware of these symptoms and identifying what triggers them, you can take proactive steps to control your asthma and minimize its impact on your life.

Recognizing Asthma Symptoms

Asthma symptoms can range from mild to severe and may occur intermittently or persistently. The classic symptoms include:

Wheezing: This is a high-pitched whistling sound that occurs when breathing, particularly during exhalation. Wheezing results from the narrowing of the airways, making it difficult for air to flow smoothly in and out of the lungs.

Shortness of Breath: This symptom can make you feel as though you can't catch your breath or are unable to get enough air into your lungs. Shortness of breath can be particularly noticeable during physical activity or at night.

Chest Tightness: Many people with asthma describe this as a feeling of pressure or squeezing in the chest. It can be uncomfortable and even painful, and it's often one of the first signs that an asthma attack may be imminent.

Coughing: A persistent cough, especially at night or early in the morning, can be a sign of asthma. The cough is typically dry and hacking, and it may worsen with exercise, cold air, or during respiratory infections.

Difficulty Sleeping: Asthma symptoms often worsen at night, leading to difficulty falling or staying asleep. This can result in daytime fatigue and reduced quality of life.

Recognizing these symptoms early and accurately can help you take appropriate action before they escalate into a full-blown asthma attack.

Identifying Asthma Triggers

Asthma triggers are factors that can provoke or worsen asthma symptoms. Triggers vary from person to person, and understanding your specific triggers is crucial for effective asthma management. Here are some common triggers and strategies to avoid or minimize exposure to them:

Allergens: Common indoor allergens include dust mites, pet dander, mold, and cockroach droppings. Outdoor allergens such as pollen from trees, grasses, and weeds can also trigger asthma. To manage these triggers, keep your home clean, use allergen-proof mattress and pillow covers, and consider using an air purifier. During high pollen seasons, keep windows closed and use air conditioning.

Irritants: Tobacco smoke, strong odors, chemical fumes, and air pollution are significant irritants that can trigger asthma symptoms. Avoid smoking or exposure to secondhand smoke, and try to stay away from strong perfumes, cleaning products, and areas with heavy air pollution.

Respiratory Infections: Colds, flu, and other respiratory infections can exacerbate asthma symptoms. Practice good hygiene, such as frequent handwashing, and consider getting annual flu vaccinations. If you feel a respiratory infection coming on, take extra precautions to manage your asthma and consult your healthcare provider if necessary.

Physical Activity: Exercise, particularly in cold or dry air, can trigger asthma symptoms. This is known as exercise-induced bronchoconstriction. Warm up gradually before exercising, use a scarf to cover your mouth and nose in cold weather, and follow your healthcare provider's advice on using a quick-relief inhaler before exercise.

Weather Conditions: Cold air, sudden temperature changes, and high humidity can trigger asthma symptoms. During cold weather, cover your mouth and nose with a scarf to warm the air you breathe. On hot, humid days, stay indoors with air conditioning if possible.

Stress and Emotions: Intense emotions such as stress, anxiety, and laughter can trigger asthma symptoms. Practice relaxation techniques such as deep breathing, meditation, and yoga to help manage stress and maintain emotional well-being.

Medications: Some medications, such as nonsteroidal anti-inflammatory drugs (NSAIDs) and beta-blockers, can trigger asthma symptoms in some people. Always inform your healthcare provider about your asthma when being prescribed new medications, and discuss any potential risks.

Keeping a symptom diary can be a powerful tool in identifying your asthma triggers. Note when and where symptoms occur, what activities you were doing, the weather conditions, and any other potential triggers you were exposed to. Over time, patterns may emerge that can help you and your healthcare provider develop a more tailored asthma management plan.

Monitoring and Managing Symptoms

Once you've recognized your asthma symptoms and identified your triggers, the next step is to monitor and manage them effectively. Here are some strategies to help you stay on top of your asthma:

Peak Flow Meters: These portable devices measure how well air moves out of your lungs. By regularly using a peak flow meter, you can detect early signs of worsening asthma and take action before symptoms become severe. Your healthcare provider can help you establish your personal best peak flow reading and set zones to indicate when you need to adjust your medication or seek medical help.

Asthma Action Plan: Work with your healthcare provider to create a personalized asthma action plan. This plan outlines daily management strategies, how to handle worsening symptoms, and when to seek emergency care. Having a clear plan can help you stay calm and in control during asthma flare-ups.

Medication Adherence: Taking your medications as prescribed is crucial for managing asthma. Long-term control medications help reduce inflammation and prevent symptoms, while quick-relief medications provide fast relief during asthma attacks. Ensure you understand how and when to use each type of medication, and never hesitate to ask your healthcare provider if you have questions.

Regular Check-ups: Regular visits to your healthcare provider can help ensure your asthma is well-managed. During these check-ups, discuss any changes in symptoms, review your medication regimen, and update your asthma action plan as needed.

Recognizing asthma symptoms and understanding your triggers are essential steps in managing asthma effectively. By staying vigilant, monitoring your condition, and working closely with your healthcare provider, you can take control of your asthma and lead a full, active life.

CHAPTER TWO

DIAGNOSIS AND TREATMENT

2.1 WORKING WITH YOUR HEALTHCARE TEAM: THE ROLE OF DOCTORS AND SPECIALISTS

Managing asthma effectively requires a collaborative effort between you and your healthcare team. Your healthcare team includes various professionals, each playing a crucial role in diagnosing, treating, and helping you manage your asthma. By understanding the roles of these healthcare providers and actively participating in your care, you can achieve better control of your asthma and improve your quality of life.

Primary Care Physicians

Your primary care physician (PCP) is often the first point of contact in managing your asthma. PCPs are trained to diagnose and treat a wide range of health conditions, including asthma. They play a pivotal role in your ongoing care, from initial diagnosis to regular monitoring and management.

Roles of Primary Care Physicians:

Initial Diagnosis: Your PCP will gather your medical history, conduct a physical examination, and order tests such as spirometry to diagnose asthma.

Developing a Treatment Plan: Based on your symptoms and test results, your PCP will create an individualized treatment plan that includes medications and lifestyle recommendations.

Prescribing Medications: Your PCP will prescribe both long-term control medications and quick-relief inhalers to manage your asthma.

Monitoring Progress: Regular check-ups with your PCP are essential to monitor your asthma control and make necessary adjustments to your treatment plan.

Referring to Specialists: If your asthma is severe or difficult to control, your PCP may refer you to a specialist for further evaluation and treatment.

Allergists and Immunologists

Allergists and immunologists specialize in diagnosing and treating allergic conditions and asthma. They are particularly helpful if your asthma is triggered by allergies or if you have other allergic conditions.

Roles of Allergists and Immunologists:

Allergy Testing: Allergists can perform tests to identify specific allergens that trigger your asthma, such as pollen, dust mites, or pet dander.

Immunotherapy: For some patients, allergists may recommend immunotherapy (allergy shots) to reduce sensitivity to allergens and improve asthma control.

Advanced Treatment Options: Allergists can provide access to specialized treatments and medications that may not be available through primary care.

Education and Counseling: Allergists offer valuable education on avoiding allergens and managing allergic triggers effectively.

Pulmonologists

Pulmonologists are specialists in lung and respiratory conditions, making them experts in managing severe or complex asthma cases. If your asthma is not well-controlled with standard treatments, a pulmonologist can provide advanced care.

Roles of Pulmonologists:

Advanced Diagnostic Testing: Pulmonologists can perform comprehensive lung function tests, imaging studies, and other diagnostic procedures to evaluate your asthma.

Specialized Treatments: They can prescribe advanced therapies, such as biologics or bronchial thermoplasty, for patients with severe asthma.

Coordinating Care: Pulmonologists work closely with other members of your healthcare team to ensure a cohesive approach to managing your asthma.

Research and Clinical Trials: They may offer access to cutting-edge research and clinical trials for new asthma treatments.

Respiratory Therapists

Respiratory therapists are trained healthcare professionals who specialize in helping patients with respiratory conditions like asthma. They provide education and support to help you manage your asthma effectively.

Roles of Respiratory Therapists:

Education on Medication Use: Respiratory therapists teach you how to use inhalers, nebulizers, and other asthma medications correctly.

Breathing Techniques: They can teach breathing exercises and techniques, such as diaphragmatic breathing and pursed-lip breathing, to improve lung function and reduce symptoms.

Asthma Action Plans: Respiratory therapists help you develop and implement personalized asthma action plans to manage symptoms and prevent attacks.

Monitoring and Support: They provide ongoing support and monitoring to help you stay on track with your asthma management plan.

Pharmacists

Pharmacists play a key role in ensuring that you understand your medications and use them safely and effectively. They are an accessible resource for medication-related questions and support.

Roles of Pharmacists:

Medication Counseling: Pharmacists can explain how to use your medications, including inhalers and spacers, and advise on potential side effects.

Drug Interactions: They check for possible interactions between your asthma medications and other drugs you may be taking.

Refill Management: Pharmacists help manage your prescription refills and ensure you have a continuous supply of your asthma medications.

Education and Support: They provide additional education on lifestyle changes, such as smoking cessation, that can improve asthma control.

Your Role in the Healthcare Team

While healthcare professionals play critical roles in managing your asthma, you are the most important member of your healthcare team. Taking an active role in your care can significantly impact your asthma control and overall well-being.

Your Responsibilities:

Communication: Be open and honest with your healthcare providers about your symptoms, triggers, and how you're feeling. Effective communication helps them tailor your treatment plan to your needs.

Adherence to Treatment: Follow your prescribed treatment plan, including taking medications as directed and using inhalers correctly. Consistency is key to keeping asthma under control.

Self-Monitoring: Use tools like peak flow meters and symptom diaries to monitor your asthma. Keeping track of your symptoms and triggers can provide valuable insights for you and your healthcare team.

Lifestyle Adjustments: Make necessary lifestyle changes to avoid triggers and improve your overall health. This may include dietary changes, regular exercise, and stress management techniques.

Education: Stay informed about asthma and its management. The more you know, the better equipped you will be to manage your condition effectively.

Building a Strong Partnership

Building a strong partnership with your healthcare team is essential for successful asthma management. Here are some tips to help you collaborate effectively with your healthcare providers:

Ask Questions: Don't hesitate to ask questions about your condition, treatment options, and any concerns you may have. Understanding your asthma and its management empowers you to take control.

Keep Appointments: Regular follow-up appointments are crucial for monitoring your asthma and making any necessary adjustments to your treatment plan.

Be Prepared: Prepare for your appointments by keeping a symptom diary, bringing a list of medications, and noting any questions or concerns you want to discuss.

Follow Up: If you experience changes in your symptoms or have difficulties with your treatment plan, reach out to your healthcare provider. Timely communication can prevent complications and ensure your asthma remains well-controlled.

Working with your healthcare team is a dynamic and ongoing process. By actively participating in your care and building strong relationships with your healthcare providers, you can achieve better asthma control and lead a healthier, more fulfilling life.

2.2 Diagnostic tools and tests for asthma

Accurate diagnosis is the cornerstone of effective asthma management. By understanding the various diagnostic tools and tests available, you can better appreciate the steps your healthcare provider takes to confirm your asthma and tailor your treatment plan. This chapter will guide you through the most common diagnostic procedures used to diagnose asthma, explaining each in a way that underscores their importance and what you can expect during the process.

Medical History and Physical Examination

The first step in diagnosing asthma typically involves a thorough review of your medical history and a physical examination. Your healthcare provider will ask about your symptoms, their frequency, and any potential triggers. This information is crucial for understanding your specific situation and guiding further testing.

Key Aspects of Medical History:

Symptom Description: Details about when your symptoms occur, how severe they are, and what seems to trigger them.

Family History: Information about any family history of asthma, allergies, or other respiratory conditions.

Personal Medical History: A review of any other medical conditions you have, including allergies and previous respiratory issues.

Lifestyle Factors: Questions about your environment, occupation, exposure to pollutants or irritants, and lifestyle habits such as smoking.

Physical Examination:

Lung Examination: Your healthcare provider will listen to your lungs with a stethoscope for signs of wheezing or other abnormal sounds.

Nasal Examination: They may check your nasal passages for signs of inflammation or other issues that could contribute to respiratory problems.

Skin Examination: Checking for signs of allergic conditions such as eczema can provide additional clues about your asthma triggers.

Spirometry

Spirometry is one of the most common and essential tests for diagnosing asthma. It measures how well your lungs are functioning by assessing the amount of air you can inhale and exhale and how quickly you can exhale.

How Spirometry Works:

Breathing Test: During a spirometry test, you will be asked to take a deep breath and then exhale forcefully into a mouthpiece connected to the spirometer.

Measurements Taken: The spirometer records two main values: Forced Vital Capacity (FVC), which is the total amount of air you can exhale after a deep breath, and

Forced Expiratory Volume in one second (FEV1), which measures how much air you can exhale in the first second.

Interpreting Results: A lower-than-normal FEV1/FVC ratio can indicate airway obstruction, a hallmark of asthma.

Spirometry is often performed before and after administering a bronchodilator, a medication that relaxes the muscles around the airways. An improvement in your spirometry results after using the bronchodilator can support an asthma diagnosis.

Peak Flow Measurement

Peak flow measurement is another tool used to diagnose and monitor asthma. It involves using a peak flow meter, a small handheld device that measures how quickly you can exhale air.

Using a Peak Flow Meter:

Taking a Reading: You will take a deep breath and blow into the mouthpiece of the peak flow meter as hard and fast as possible.

Recording Results: The meter provides a reading, known as peak expiratory flow (PEF), which you will record. This process is typically repeated several times to ensure accuracy.

Monitoring Changes: Regular peak flow measurements can help you and your healthcare provider monitor your asthma control over time and identify patterns or triggers.

Methacholine Challenge Test

If your asthma symptoms and spirometry results are inconclusive, your healthcare provider may recommend a methacholine challenge test. Methacholine is a substance that, when inhaled, can cause airway constriction in individuals with asthma.

How the Test Works:

Inhalation: You will inhale increasing concentrations of methacholine aerosol while your lung function is monitored using spirometry.

Response: A significant decrease in lung function (FEV1) after inhaling methacholine indicates hyperreactive airways, which is characteristic of asthma.

Reversibility: After the test, you will receive a bronchodilator to reverse the effects of methacholine, ensuring your airways return to normal.

Exhaled Nitric Oxide Test (FeNO)

The exhaled nitric oxide test measures the level of nitric oxide in your breath, which can indicate airway inflammation—a common feature of asthma.

Test Procedure:

Breathing Test: You will breathe into a mouthpiece connected to the nitric oxide analyzer, which measures the concentration of nitric oxide in your exhaled breath.

Interpreting Results: Higher levels of exhaled nitric oxide suggest airway inflammation and can support an asthma diagnosis, particularly if you have allergic or eosinophilic asthma.

Allergy Testing

Since allergies often play a significant role in asthma, allergy testing can help identify specific allergens that trigger your symptoms. There are two main types of allergy tests: skin tests and blood tests.

Skin Prick Test:

Procedure: Small amounts of suspected allergens are applied to your skin, usually on your forearm or back. The skin is then pricked to allow the allergens to enter.

Reaction: If you are allergic to a substance, you will develop a small raised bump at the test site, usually within 15-20 minutes.

Blood Test:

Procedure: A blood sample is taken to measure the level of specific antibodies (IgE) to various allergens.

Results: Elevated levels of IgE antibodies suggest an allergic response to particular substances.

Chest X-Ray and CT scan

While not routinely used for diagnosing asthma, chest X-rays or CT scans may be performed to rule out other conditions that can mimic asthma symptoms, such as infections or structural abnormalities in the lungs.

Imaging Tests:

Chest X-Ray: Provides a basic image of your lungs and can help detect issues like infections or large obstructions.

CT scan: Offers a more detailed view of the lungs and can identify smaller or more complex issues that may not be visible on a standard X-ray.

Sputum Eosinophils

This test examines the presence of eosinophils, a type of white blood cell, in your sputum (mucus you cough up). Elevated levels of eosinophils can indicate eosinophilic asthma, which is often associated with severe asthma and may require specialized treatments.

Procedure:

Sample Collection: You will provide a sample of your sputum, which is then analyzed in a laboratory.

Results: High levels of eosinophils suggest inflammation and can help tailor your treatment plan.

Exercise and Cold Air Challenge Tests

These tests help identify exercise-induced asthma or asthma triggered by cold air. They involve controlled exposure to exercise or cold air while monitoring your lung function.

Exercise Challenge Test:

Procedure: You will perform physical activity, usually on a treadmill or stationary bike, while your lung function is monitored before and after exercise.

Results: A significant decrease in lung function post-exercise can indicate exercise-induced asthma.

Cold Air Challenge Test:

Procedure: You will inhale cold air, often combined with a controlled physical activity, while your lung function is monitored.

Results: A drop in lung function after exposure to cold air can indicate cold air-induced asthma.

Diagnosing asthma involves a combination of medical history, physical examination, and various diagnostic tests to accurately identify the condition and its triggers. Understanding these diagnostic tools and procedures can help you navigate the diagnostic process with confidence and actively participate in your care. With a clear diagnosis, you and your healthcare team can develop an effective treatment plan tailored to your specific needs, setting you on the path to better asthma management and improved quality of life.

2.3 Understanding your personalized treatment plan

Asthma is a highly individualized condition, meaning that what works for one person may not necessarily work for another. This is why creating a personalized treatment plan is essential. A well-crafted plan addresses your specific triggers, symptoms, and lifestyle, ensuring that you can manage your asthma effectively and live a full, active life. Let's explore the key components of a personalized asthma treatment plan and how each part contributes to managing your condition.

The Foundation of Your Treatment Plan: Assessment and Goals

The first step in developing a personalized treatment plan is a thorough assessment by your healthcare provider. This includes understanding the severity of your asthma, identifying your specific triggers, and determining your overall health and lifestyle needs. The primary goals of your treatment plan will be to:

- Prevent chronic and troublesome symptoms such as coughing and shortness of breath
- Maintain normal lung function and activity levels
- Prevent asthma attacks and emergency room visits
- Minimize the need for quick-relief medications

- Address any concerns or questions you may have about your asthma and its management

Long-Term Control Medications

Long-term control medications are taken daily to maintain control of persistent asthma and prevent symptoms. These medications are a cornerstone of your asthma treatment plan and are necessary even when you feel fine, as they help prevent symptoms from returning.

Types of Long-Term Control Medications:

1. Inhaled Corticosteroids:

- Function: Reduce inflammation in the airways, making them less sensitive and less likely to react to triggers.
- Common Options: Fluticasone (Flovent), Budesonide (Pulmicort), Beclomethasone (Qvar).
- Usage: Usually taken once or twice daily using an inhaler.

2. Long-Acting Beta-Agonists (LABAs):

- Function: Help relax the muscles around the airways and keep them open for up to 12 hours.

- Common Options: Salmeterol (Serevent), Formoterol (Foradil).

- Usage: Often combined with inhaled corticosteroids in a single inhaler.

3. Leukotriene Modifiers:

- Function: Block the action of leukotrienes, chemicals in the immune system that cause inflammation and mucus production.

- Common Options: Montelukast (Singulair), Zafirlukast (Accolate).

- Usage: Taken orally, usually once daily.

4. Mast Cell Stabilizers:

- Function: Prevent the release of inflammatory chemicals from mast cells.

- Common Options: Cromolyn sodium (Intal), Nedocromil (Tilade).

- Usage: Inhaled, used less frequently than other long-term medications.

5. Theophylline:

- Function: Helps open the airways by relaxing the muscles around them.

- Common Options: Theophylline (Theo-24, Elixophyllin).

- Usage: Taken orally, requires regular blood tests to monitor levels.

Quick-Relief Medications

Quick-relief, or rescue, medications provide immediate relief from asthma symptoms and are essential for managing sudden asthma attacks. These medications work rapidly to relax tight muscles around the airways, making it easier to breathe.

Types of Quick-Relief Medications:

1. Short-Acting Beta-Agonists (SABAs):

- Function: Quickly relax the muscles around the airways.

- Common Options: Albuterol (ProAir, Ventolin), Levalbuterol (Xopenex).
- Usage: Used as needed for rapid symptom relief.

1. **Anticholinergics:**

- Function: Help relax the muscles around the airways and reduce mucus production.
- Common Options: Ipratropium (Atrovent).
- Usage: Can be used in combination with SABAs during an asthma attack.

2. **Systemic Corticosteroids:**

- Function: Reduce airway inflammation during severe asthma episodes.
- Common Options: Prednisone, Methylprednisolone.
- Usage: Taken orally or intravenously, usually for short periods due to side effects.

Identifying and Avoiding Triggers

A critical aspect of your treatment plan involves identifying and managing asthma triggers. Triggers can vary widely among individuals, so it's essential to pinpoint what specifically affects you.

Common Asthma Triggers:

- Allergens: Pollen, dust mites, pet dander, mold.
- Irritants: Smoke, strong odors, air pollution.
- Respiratory Infections: Colds, flu, sinus infections.
- Physical Activity: Exercise-induced asthma.
- Weather Conditions: Cold air, changes in humidity.
- Stress and Emotions: Anxiety, stress, laughter.

Strategies to Avoid Triggers:

Environmental Control: Use air purifiers, maintain a clean home, use allergen-proof covers for bedding.

Personal Habits: Avoid smoking, reduce exposure to secondhand smoke, manage stress through relaxation techniques.

Health Management: Get vaccinated against flu and pneumonia, practice good hygiene to avoid infections.

Monitoring Your Asthma

Regular monitoring of your asthma is essential to ensure your treatment plan is effective and to make necessary adjustments. This involves both self-monitoring and regular check-ups with your healthcare provider.

Self-Monitoring Tools:

Peak Flow Meters: Measure your peak expiratory flow rate (PEFR) to detect changes in your lung function.

Asthma Diaries: Record your symptoms, medication use, and peak flow readings to identify patterns and triggers.

Smartphone Apps: Use apps designed to track asthma symptoms and medication use, providing real-time data to share with your healthcare provider.

Regular Check-Ups:

Frequency: Initially, you may need frequent visits to your healthcare provider to adjust your treatment plan. Once your asthma is well-controlled, check-ups may be less frequent, such as every three to six months.

Assessments: Your provider will assess your symptom control, review your medication technique, and adjust your treatment plan as needed.

Asthma Action Plan

An asthma action plan is a written document that outlines how to manage your asthma daily and what steps to take during an asthma attack. This plan is personalized to your specific needs and should be developed in collaboration with your healthcare provider.

Components of an Asthma Action Plan:

Daily Management: Instructions on your daily medications and strategies to avoid triggers.

Symptom Monitoring: Guidelines on how to recognize worsening symptoms and when to use your quick-relief inhaler.

Emergency Steps: Clear instructions on what to do during an asthma attack, including when to seek emergency medical care.

Zones in an Asthma Action Plan:

Green Zone: Your asthma is well-controlled. You have no symptoms and can perform usual activities.

Yellow Zone: Your asthma is getting worse. You may have symptoms like coughing, wheezing, or shortness of breath. Follow the steps in your action plan to get back to the green zone.

Red Zone: Your asthma is severe. You have significant symptoms and need to take immediate action, which may include using quick-relief medications and seeking emergency medical care.

Education and Support

Education is a vital part of managing asthma. Understanding your condition, knowing how to use your medications correctly, and being aware of your triggers empower you to take control of your asthma.

Educational Resources:

Healthcare Providers: Utilize the knowledge and experience of your doctors, nurses, and respiratory therapists.

Support Groups: Join asthma support groups, either in-person or online, to share experiences and tips with others who have asthma.

Educational Materials: Read books, brochures, and reputable websites dedicated to asthma education.

Creating and following a personalized asthma treatment plan is essential for managing your condition effectively. By working closely with your healthcare team, understanding your medications, identifying and avoiding triggers, and regularly monitoring your asthma, you can achieve better control and enjoy a healthier, more active life.

2.3 Medication options and their uses

Asthma management often hinges on the effective use of medications tailored to your specific needs.

Understanding the variety of medication options and their specific uses can empower you to manage your asthma effectively and improve your quality of life. This chapter will explore the different types of asthma medications, how they work, and how they fit into your overall treatment plan.

Long-Term Control Medications

Long-term control medications, also known as maintenance or controller medications, are used daily to keep asthma under control. They help reduce inflammation, prevent symptoms, and minimize the risk of asthma attacks. Even if you feel well, it is crucial to take these medications regularly as prescribed.

1. Inhaled Corticosteroids (ICS)

Inhaled corticosteroids are the most commonly prescribed long-term control medications. They work by reducing inflammation in the airways, making them less sensitive and less likely to react to triggers.

- How They Work: Inhaled corticosteroids reduce swelling and mucus production in the airways, which helps prevent asthma symptoms and improve lung function.

- Common Medications: Fluticasone (Flovent), Budesonide (Pulmicort), Beclomethasone (Qvar), Mometasone (Asmanex).

- Usage: Typically taken once or twice daily using an inhaler. It's important to rinse your mouth after using ICS to prevent side effects like oral thrush.

2. Long-Acting Beta-Agonists (LABAs)

LABAs are bronchodilators that help keep the airways open for up to 12 hours. They are often used in combination with inhaled corticosteroids.

- How They Work: LABAs relax the muscles around the airways, helping to keep them open and making breathing easier.

- Common Medications: Salmeterol (Serevent), Formoterol (Foradil).

- Usage: Used twice daily, usually in combination with an inhaled corticosteroid. They should not be used as monotherapy for asthma.

3. Combination Inhalers

Combination inhalers contain both an inhaled corticosteroid and a long-acting beta-agonist. They simplify treatment by delivering both medications in a single inhaler.

- How They Work: Provide the anti-inflammatory benefits of corticosteroids and the bronchodilation of LABAs in one device.

- Common Medications: Fluticasone/Salmeterol (Advair), Budesonide/Formoterol (Symbicort), Mometasone/Formoterol (Dulera).

- Usage: Typically used twice daily. They help improve adherence to medication regimens by combining two medications into one.

4. Leukotriene Modifiers

Leukotriene modifiers block the action of leukotrienes, chemicals in the immune system that cause inflammation and mucus production.

- How They Work: These medications reduce inflammation, decrease mucus secretion, and prevent airway constriction.
- Common Medications: Montelukast (Singulair), Zafirlukast (Accolate), Zileuton (Zyflo).
- Usage: Taken orally once daily. They are particularly useful for patients with allergic asthma.

5. Mast Cell Stabilizers

Mast cell stabilizers prevent the release of inflammatory chemicals from mast cells, which helps prevent asthma symptoms.

- How They Work: These medications help prevent airway inflammation and reduce symptoms triggered by allergens or exercise.

- Common Medications: Cromolyn sodium (Intal), Nedocromil (Tilade).

- Usage: Inhaled, typically used two to four times daily. They are less commonly prescribed than other long-term medications.

6. Theophylline

Theophylline is a bronchodilator that helps open the airways by relaxing the muscles around them.

- How It Works: Theophylline relaxes bronchial muscles, reduces airway responsiveness to allergens and irritants, and increases the contraction of the diaphragm, making breathing easier.

- Common Medications: Theophylline (Theo-24, Elixophyllin).

- Usage: Taken orally, usually once or twice daily. Regular blood tests are required to monitor therapeutic levels and avoid toxicity.

Quick-Relief Medications

Quick-relief, or rescue, medications provide immediate relief from asthma symptoms and are essential for managing sudden asthma attacks. These medications work rapidly to relax tight muscles around the airways, making it easier to breathe.

1. Short-Acting Beta-Agonists (SABAs)

SABAs are the most commonly used rescue medications. They provide quick relief from acute asthma symptoms and are often referred to as "rescue inhalers."

- How They Work: SABAs quickly relax the muscles around the airways, making it easier to breathe within minutes.

- Common Medications: Albuterol (ProAir, Ventolin), Levalbuterol (Xopenex).

- Usage: Used as needed for rapid symptom relief. They are typically inhaled using a metered-dose inhaler (MDI) or a nebulizer.

2. Anticholinergics

Anticholinergics help relax the muscles around the airways and reduce mucus production. They are sometimes used in combination with SABAs during an asthma attack.

- How They Work: These medications block the action of acetylcholine, a chemical that causes airway muscles to constrict and mucus glands to secrete.
- Common Medications: Ipratropium (Atrovent), Tiotropium (Spiriva).
- Usage: Inhaled using an MDI or nebulizer. They are often used as an add-on therapy for severe asthma exacerbations.

3. Systemic Corticosteroids

Systemic corticosteroids are used for severe asthma attacks that do not respond to other treatments. They help reduce inflammation throughout the body.

- How They Work: These medications reduce inflammation in the airways, making it easier to breathe.
- Common Medications: Prednisone, Methylprednisolone (Medrol).
- Usage: Taken orally or intravenously for short periods due to potential side effects.

Biologic Therapies

Biologic therapies are a newer class of medications used to treat severe asthma that is not well controlled with standard treatments. They target specific molecules involved in the inflammatory process.

1. Anti-IgE Therapy

Anti-IgE therapy targets immunoglobulin E (IgE), an antibody that plays a key role in allergic asthma.

- How It Works: This therapy prevents IgE from binding to mast cells and basophils, reducing the release of inflammatory chemicals.
- Common Medications: Omalizumab (Xolair).

- Usage: Administered via injection every 2-4 weeks. It is used for patients with moderate to severe allergic asthma.

2. Anti-IL-5 Therapy

Anti-IL-5 therapy targets interleukin-5 (IL-5), a cytokine involved in the activation and survival of eosinophils, a type of white blood cell that contributes to asthma inflammation.

- How It Works: These medications reduce the number of eosinophils in the blood and airways, decreasing inflammation.
- Common Medications: Mepolizumab (Nucala), Reslizumab (Cinqair), Benralizumab (Fasenra).
- Usage: Administered via injection or intravenous infusion. Used for patients with severe eosinophilic asthma.

3. Anti-IL-4 and Anti-IL-13 Therapy

These therapies target interleukins 4 and 13, cytokines that play a role in the allergic inflammatory process.

- How They Work: These medications block the action of IL-4 and IL-13, reducing airway inflammation and mucus production.

- Common Medications: Dupilumab (Dupixent).

- Usage: Administered via injection every 2 weeks. Used for patients with moderate to severe asthma with an allergic component.

Immunotherapy

Immunotherapy, also known as allergy shots, is used to reduce sensitivity to allergens over time. It involves gradually increasing doses of the allergen to build tolerance.

How It Works:

- Gradual Exposure: Small doses of the allergen are injected over a period of time, with doses gradually increasing.

- Immune Response: Over time, your immune system becomes less sensitive to the allergen, reducing allergy and asthma symptoms.

- Usage: Typically involves a build-up phase of weekly injections followed by a maintenance phase of monthly injections.

Navigating the world of asthma medications can be complex, but understanding the different options and their uses is vital for effective management. Long-term control medications help maintain stable asthma control, while quick-relief medications provide essential support during flare-ups. Newer biologic therapies offer hope for those with severe asthma not well-managed by traditional treatments. By working closely with your healthcare provider and adhering to your personalized treatment plan, you can achieve better control of your asthma and lead a healthier, more active life.

CHAPTER THREE

PARTNERING WITH YOUR BODY

3.1 MONITORING YOUR ASTHMA: PEAK FLOW METERS AND SYMPTOM TRACKING

Effectively monitoring your asthma is crucial for maintaining control of your condition and preventing exacerbations. In this chapter, we will explore the importance of monitoring your asthma symptoms and lung function using peak flow meters and symptom tracking. These tools empower you to take an active role in managing your asthma and provide valuable insights into your overall lung health.

The Role of Monitoring in Asthma Management

Monitoring your asthma involves regularly assessing your symptoms, peak expiratory flow (PEF) or peak flow, and medication use. By keeping track of these factors over time, you and your healthcare provider can identify patterns, recognize triggers, and adjust your treatment plan as needed to achieve optimal asthma control.

Symptom Monitoring:

Pay attention to common asthma symptoms such as coughing, wheezing, shortness of breath, and chest tightness.

Keep a journal or diary to record the frequency, severity, and duration of your symptoms.

Note any triggers or environmental factors that may exacerbate your asthma symptoms.

Peak Flow Monitoring

Peak flow meters are handheld devices that measure the maximum speed at which you can expel air from your lungs.

Regular peak flow measurements can help assess changes in your lung function and detect asthma flare-ups before symptoms worsen.

Your healthcare provider may provide you with a personalized peak flow management plan based on your individual peak flow readings.

Using Peak Flow Meters

Peak flow meters are simple yet powerful tools for monitoring your asthma and tracking changes in your lung function over time. Here's how to use a peak flow meter effectively:

Select the Right Peak Flow Meter: Choose a peak flow meter that is appropriate for your age and lung capacity. There are different types of peak flow meters available, including handheld devices and portable electronic meters.

Establish Your Personal Best Peak Flow: Measure your peak flow when your asthma is well-controlled to establish your personal best peak flow. This baseline value serves as a reference point for monitoring changes in your lung function.

Follow a Consistent Testing Routine: Measure your peak flow at the same time each day, preferably in the morning before taking asthma medications. Stand up straight and take a deep breath before performing the test.

Record Your Peak Flow Readings: Keep a record of your peak flow measurements in a peak flow diary or asthma action plan. Note any symptoms or triggers that may have influenced your readings.

Interpret Your Peak Flow Readings: Compare your current peak flow readings to your personal best peak flow and the predicted values for someone of your age, height, and gender. Your healthcare provider can help you interpret your peak flow readings and adjust your treatment plan accordingly.

Symptom Tracking

In addition to monitoring your peak flow, it's essential to track your asthma symptoms regularly. Symptom tracking helps you identify patterns, triggers, and trends in your asthma control. Here are some tips for effective symptom tracking:

Keep a Symptom Diary: Record any asthma symptoms you experience, including coughing, wheezing, shortness of breath, and chest tightness. Note the time of day, duration, and severity of each symptom.

Identify Triggers: Pay attention to factors that may trigger your asthma symptoms, such as allergens, exercise, weather changes, respiratory infections, and stress. By identifying your triggers, you can take steps to avoid or minimize exposure to them.

Use Symptom Rating Scales: Rate the severity of your symptoms using a numerical or descriptive scale, such as mild, moderate, or severe. This allows you to track changes in your symptoms over time and communicate effectively with your healthcare provider.

Monitor Medication Use: Keep track of the medications you use to manage your asthma, including both long-term control medications and quick-relief medications. Note any changes in your medication regimen and how they affect your asthma control.

Incorporating Monitoring into Your Asthma Management Plan

Monitoring your asthma should be an integral part of your asthma management plan. By regularly tracking your symptoms and peak flow measurements, you can:

- Identify early warning signs of worsening asthma control.

- Determine the effectiveness of your current treatment plan.

- Make informed decisions about adjusting your medication regimen.

- Communicate effectively with your healthcare provider about your asthma control and treatment goals.

Monitoring your asthma using peak flow meters and symptom tracking is a valuable tool for achieving and maintaining optimal asthma control. By actively participating in your asthma management and staying vigilant about changes in your lung function and symptoms, you can take proactive steps to prevent asthma flare-ups and enjoy a better quality of life.

3.2 Understanding long-term control and rescue medications

In the management of asthma, medications play a crucial role in controlling symptoms, preventing exacerbations, and improving overall lung function. Long-term control medications are used daily to manage underlying inflammation and keep asthma symptoms at bay, while rescue medications provide rapid relief during acute asthma attacks. Let's delve into the different types of long-term control and rescue medications, how they work, and when they are used in asthma management.

Long-Term Control Medications

Long-term control medications are the cornerstone of asthma management for individuals with persistent asthma. These medications work by reducing inflammation in the airways and preventing symptoms from occurring.

Inhaled Corticosteroids (ICS):

How They Work: Inhaled corticosteroids reduce inflammation in the airways, making them less sensitive and less likely to react to triggers.

Common Medications: Fluticasone (Flovent), Budesonide (Pulmicort), Beclomethasone (Qvar).

Usage: Typically taken once or twice daily using an inhaler.

Long-Acting Beta-Agonists (LABAs):

How They Work: LABAs help relax the muscles around the airways, keeping them open for up to 12 hours.

Common Medications: Salmeterol (Serevent), Formoterol (Foradil).

Usage: Often combined with inhaled corticosteroids in a single inhaler for twice-daily dosing.

Leukotriene Modifiers:

How They Work: Leukotriene modifiers block the action of leukotrienes, chemicals in the immune system that cause inflammation and mucus production.

Common Medications: Montelukast (Singulair), Zafirlukast (Accolate).

Usage: Taken orally once daily.

Mast Cell Stabilizers:

How They Work: Mast cell stabilizers prevent the release of inflammatory chemicals from mast cells.

Common Medications: Cromolyn sodium (Intal), Nedocromil (Tilade).

Usage: Inhaled, typically used two to four times daily.

Theophylline:

How It Works: Theophylline helps open the airways by relaxing the muscles around them.

Common Medications: Theophylline (Theo-24, Elixophyllin).

Usage: Taken orally once or twice daily, requires regular blood tests to monitor levels.

Rescue Medications

Rescue medications, also known as quick-relief medications, provide rapid relief of asthma symptoms during acute exacerbations or flare-ups. These medications work quickly to relax the muscles around the airways, making it easier to breathe.

Short-Acting Beta-Agonists (SABAs):

How They Work: SABAs quickly relax the muscles around the airways, providing rapid relief of asthma symptoms within minutes.

Common Medications: Albuterol (ProAir, Ventolin), Levalbuterol (Xopenex).

Usage: Used as needed for immediate symptom relief.

Anticholinergics:

How They Work: Anticholinergics help relax the muscles around the airways and reduce mucus production.

Common Medications: Ipratropium (Atrovent).

Usage: Inhaled, often used in combination with SABAs during asthma exacerbations.

Systemic Corticosteroids:

How They Work: Systemic corticosteroids reduce inflammation throughout the body, including the airways.

Common Medications: Prednisone, Methylprednisolone.

Usage: Taken orally or intravenously for short periods during severe asthma exacerbations.

Understanding the Role of Each Medication

Long-term control medications are used to manage underlying inflammation and prevent asthma symptoms from occurring on a daily basis. They are taken regularly, even when symptoms are well-controlled, to maintain stable asthma control and prevent exacerbations.

Rescue medications, on the other hand, are used as needed to provide rapid relief of asthma symptoms during acute exacerbations or flare-ups. They should not be used as a long-term solution for managing asthma and do not address the underlying inflammation in the airways.

Creating a Personalized Asthma Management Plan

Effective asthma management involves creating a personalized treatment plan in collaboration with your healthcare provider. This plan should include both long-term control medications to manage underlying inflammation and prevent symptoms, as well as rescue medications to provide rapid relief during acute exacerbations.

By understanding the role of each medication in your asthma management plan and adhering to your prescribed treatment regimen, you can achieve better asthma control, reduce the frequency and severity of exacerbations, and improve your overall quality of life.

3.3 The importance of medication adherence and technique

Ensuring proper adherence to your asthma medication regimen and mastering the correct inhaler technique are essential components of effective asthma management. In this section of this chapter, we will explore why medication adherence and technique matter, how they can impact your asthma control, and practical strategies for improving both aspects of your treatment.

Understanding Medication Adherence

Medication adherence refers to the extent to which patients take their medications as prescribed by their healthcare provider. It encompasses not only taking the correct dose of medication but also following the prescribed schedule and using the correct technique when administering inhalers or other asthma medications.

Why Medication Adherence Matters:

Optimal Asthma Control: Adhering to your prescribed medication regimen is crucial for achieving and maintaining optimal asthma control. Skipping doses or using medications inconsistently can lead to increased symptoms, exacerbations, and decreased lung function over time.

Prevention of Exacerbations: Consistent medication adherence helps prevent asthma exacerbations and reduces the need for emergency medical care or hospitalizations.

Improvement in Quality of Life: By effectively managing your asthma symptoms through medication adherence, you can enjoy a better quality of life with fewer limitations on daily activities.

Challenges to Medication Adherence

Despite the importance of medication adherence, many individuals with asthma face challenges that can affect their ability to adhere to their prescribed treatment regimen. Common barriers to adherence include:

Forgetfulness: Forgetting to take medications regularly or at the correct times.

Cost of Medications: Financial constraints or lack of insurance coverage for asthma medications.

Misunderstanding of Instructions: Difficulty understanding medication instructions or concerns about potential side effects.

Inconvenience: Difficulty incorporating medication administration into daily routines or travel plans.

Perceived Lack of Need: Feeling well and believing that medications are unnecessary, especially during periods of symptom remission.

Strategics for Improving Medication Adherence

Overcoming barriers to medication adherence requires a proactive approach and the implementation of practical strategies tailored to individual needs. Here are some tips for improving medication adherence:

Educate Yourself: Take the time to understand the importance of your asthma medications and how they work to manage your symptoms and prevent exacerbations. Ask your healthcare provider any questions you may have about your treatment regimen.

Develop a Routine: Incorporate medication administration into your daily routine by taking medications at the same time each day. Use reminders such as alarms, pill organizers, or smartphone apps to help you remember.

Communicate with Your Healthcare Provider: Be open and honest with your healthcare provider about any challenges or concerns you may have regarding your medications. They can work with you to address these issues and find solutions that fit your lifestyle.

Seek Support: Lean on friends, family members, or support groups for encouragement and accountability in adhering to your medication regimen. Having a support system can make a significant difference in staying motivated and committed to your treatment plan.

Mastering Inhaler Technique

In addition to medication adherence, mastering the correct technique for using inhalers is crucial for ensuring the optimal delivery of medication to your lungs. Proper inhaler technique maximizes the effectiveness of asthma medications and reduces the risk of side effects.

Why Inhaler Technique Matters:

Optimal Medication Delivery: Using the correct inhaler technique ensures that the medication reaches your lungs where it is needed to control asthma symptoms and inflammation.

Minimization of Side Effects: Proper inhaler technique reduces the risk of side effects such as oral thrush or hoarseness, which can occur when medications are not administered correctly.

Enhancement of Asthma Control: By mastering inhaler technique, you can improve the efficacy of your asthma medications and achieve better asthma control with lower doses.

Common Mistakes in Inhaler Technique

Despite the importance of proper inhaler technique, many individuals with asthma struggle to use their inhalers correctly. Common mistakes in inhaler technique include:

Improper Breath Coordination: Failing to coordinate inhalation with actuation, resulting in inadequate medication delivery to the lungs.

Failure to Breathe Out Fully: Forgetting to exhale fully before inhaling medication, which can lead to poor medication deposition in the lungs.

Insufficient Inhalation Force: Not inhaling forcefully enough to ensure proper medication dispersion throughout the lungs.

Incorrect Spacer Use: Using a metered-dose inhaler without a spacer or failing to use a spacer correctly, resulting in decreased medication delivery to the lungs.

Strategies for Improving Inhaler Technique

Improving inhaler technique requires practice, patience, and guidance from your healthcare provider. Here are some tips for mastering inhaler technique:

Receive Proper Training: Ask your healthcare provider to demonstrate the correct technique for using your inhaler and observe closely to ensure you understand the steps involved.

Practice Regularly: Practice using your inhaler technique in front of a mirror or with a spacer device to ensure proper coordination of inhalation and medication actuation.

Use Spacer Devices: If prescribed, use a spacer device with your metered-dose inhaler to improve medication delivery to the lungs and reduce the risk of side effects.

Seek Feedback: Ask your healthcare provider to observe your inhaler technique and provide feedback on areas for improvement. They can offer personalized tips and strategies to help you master the correct technique.

Medication adherence and technique are essential components of effective asthma management. By adhering to your prescribed medication regimen and mastering the correct inhaler technique, you can achieve better asthma control, reduce the risk of exacerbations, and improve your overall quality of life. Remember to communicate openly with your healthcare provider about any challenges or concerns you may have regarding your asthma medications, and seek support from your support system to stay motivated and committed to your treatment plan.

CHAPTER FOUR

BUILDING A HEALTHY LIFESTYLE WITH ASTHMA

4.1 IDENTIFYING AND AVOIDING COMMON ASTHMA TRIGGERS

Understanding and managing asthma triggers is essential for maintaining control over your asthma symptoms and reducing the risk of exacerbations. In this chapter, we will explore common asthma triggers, how they can affect your asthma control, and practical strategies for identifying and avoiding them in your daily life.

What Are Asthma Triggers?

Asthma triggers are substances or environmental factors that can exacerbate asthma symptoms or lead to asthma attacks in individuals with asthma. These triggers vary from person to person, and what may trigger asthma symptoms in one individual may not affect another. By identifying and avoiding your specific asthma triggers, you can reduce the frequency and severity of asthma symptoms and improve your overall asthma control.

Common Asthma Triggers

1. Allergens:

- Pollen: Pollen from trees, grasses, and weeds can trigger asthma symptoms, particularly during allergy seasons.

- Dust Mites: Dust mites are tiny insects that thrive in bedding, upholstered furniture, and carpets and can trigger allergic reactions in individuals with asthma.

- Mold: Mold spores found in damp and humid environments, such as bathrooms, basements, and air conditioning units, can exacerbate asthma symptoms.

- Pet Dander: Proteins found in the skin, saliva, and urine of pets can trigger asthma symptoms in individuals allergic to animals.

2. Environmental Irritants:

- Tobacco Smoke: Exposure to tobacco smoke, whether firsthand or secondhand, can worsen asthma symptoms and increase the risk of asthma attacks.

- Air Pollution: Outdoor air pollutants such as vehicle emissions, industrial pollutants, and particulate matter can irritate the airways and exacerbate asthma symptoms.

- Strong Odors: Perfumes, household cleaning products, and other strong odors can trigger asthma symptoms in sensitive individuals.

3. Respiratory Infections:

Viruses: Respiratory infections caused by viruses such as the common cold, flu, and respiratory syncytial virus (RSV) can exacerbate asthma symptoms and increase the risk of asthma attacks.

4. Physical Activity:

Exercise: Intense physical activity or exercise can trigger asthma symptoms, particularly in individuals with exercise-induced asthma.

5. Weather Changes:

Cold Air: Breathing in cold, dry air can irritate the airways and trigger asthma symptoms, especially during winter months.

Humidity: High humidity levels can promote the growth of mold and dust mites, leading to increased asthma symptoms in sensitive individuals.

Strategies for Identifying and Avoiding Asthma Triggers

1. Keep a Trigger Diary: Keep track of your asthma symptoms and potential triggers in a diary or journal. Note any patterns or trends in your symptoms and the environmental factors or activities that may have triggered them.

2. Undergo Allergy Testing: Consider undergoing allergy testing to identify specific allergens that may be triggering your asthma symptoms. Allergy testing can help you develop a targeted approach to avoiding allergens in your environment.

3. Create an Asthma-Safe Home Environment:

- Dust Control: Use allergen-proof mattress and pillow covers, wash bedding regularly in hot water, and vacuum carpets and upholstered furniture frequently to reduce dust mite exposure.

- Mold Prevention: Keep indoor humidity levels below 50%, fix any leaks or water damage promptly, and clean bathrooms and other damp areas regularly to prevent mold growth.

- Pet Management: If you have pets, consider keeping them out of bedrooms and other areas where you spend a lot of time. Bathe pets regularly and vacuum pet hair and dander from carpets and furniture.

4. Avoid Tobacco Smoke and Air Pollution:

Quit Smoking: If you smoke, quit smoking to improve your asthma control and reduce the risk of asthma exacerbations.

Avoid Secondhand Smoke: Avoid exposure to secondhand smoke from others, and encourage family members and visitors to smoke outside of the home.

Monitor Air Quality: Check local air quality reports and avoid outdoor activities on days when air pollution levels are high.

5. Manage Respiratory Infections:

Practice Good Hygiene: Wash your hands frequently with soap and water, avoid touching your face, and cover your mouth and nose when coughing or sneezing to reduce the risk of respiratory infections.

6. Use Asthma Medications as Prescribed:

Long-Term Control Medications: Take your long-term control medications regularly as prescribed by your healthcare provider to prevent asthma symptoms and exacerbations.

Rescue Medications: Have your rescue inhaler on hand at all times and use it as needed for rapid relief of asthma symptoms.

Identifying and avoiding common asthma triggers is essential for achieving and maintaining optimal asthma control. By understanding your individual asthma triggers and taking proactive steps to minimize exposure to them, you can reduce the frequency and severity of asthma symptoms, prevent asthma exacerbations, and improve your overall quality of life.

4. 2 Managing indoor allergens: dust mites, mold, and pet dander

In our homes, we encounter a multitude of potential asthma triggers, many of which are invisible to the naked eye. Dust mites, mold, and pet dander are among the most common indoor allergens that can exacerbate asthma symptoms and lead to respiratory distress. In this chapter, we will transverse practical strategies for identifying, reducing, and managing these indoor allergens to create a healthier indoor environment and improve asthma control.

Dust Mites: The Tiny Culprits

Dust mites are microscopic insects that thrive in warm, humid environments, such as bedding, upholstered furniture, and carpeting. These tiny creatures feed on dead skin cells shed by humans and pets, and their feces contain proteins that can trigger allergic reactions in sensitive individuals. Here's how to tackle dust mites in your home:

Encase Mattresses and Pillows: Use allergen-proof covers for mattresses and pillows to create a barrier against dust mites and their allergens.

Wash Bedding Regularly: Wash bedding, including sheets, pillowcases, and blankets, in hot water (130°F or higher) weekly to kill dust mites and remove allergens.

Vacuum Frequently: Vacuum carpets, rugs, and upholstered furniture regularly using a vacuum cleaner equipped with a HEPA filter to trap dust mites and allergens.

Reduce Humidity: Maintain indoor humidity levels below 50% to inhibit dust mite growth. Use a dehumidifier in damp areas such as basements and bathrooms if necessary.

Mold: The Hidden Threat

Mold is a type of fungus that thrives in damp, humid environments and can be found both indoors and outdoors. Mold spores can become airborne and trigger asthma symptoms when inhaled by sensitive individuals. To combat mold in your home:

Fix Leaks and Moisture Issues: Promptly repair any leaks or water damage in your home, including plumbing leaks, roof leaks, and condensation buildup.

Ventilate Moist Areas: Use exhaust fans in bathrooms and kitchens to vent moisture outside, and open windows to increase ventilation and airflow in humid areas.

Clean and Remove Mold: Clean moldy surfaces with a solution of water and detergent, and promptly remove and replace any moldy materials such as carpeting or ceiling tiles.

Pet Dander: Furry Friends, Potential Triggers

Pet dander consists of tiny flecks of skin shed by pets such as cats, dogs, and rodents, as well as proteins found in their saliva and urine. These allergens can become airborne and settle on surfaces throughout the home, triggering asthma symptoms in susceptible individuals. Here's how to manage pet dander:

Establish Pet-Free Zones: Designate certain areas of your home, such as bedrooms or other sleeping areas, as pet-free zones to minimize exposure to pet dander while you sleep.

Bathe Pets Regularly: Bathe pets regularly to reduce the amount of dander and allergens they shed. Use pet-friendly shampoos and grooming products recommended by your veterinarian.

Clean Surfaces Frequently: Wipe down surfaces such as countertops, floors, and furniture regularly to remove pet dander and allergens. Use a vacuum cleaner with a HEPA filter to effectively trap pet hair and dander.

Managing indoor allergens such as dust mites, mold, and pet dander is essential for individuals with asthma to reduce the frequency and severity of asthma symptoms and improve overall asthma control. By implementing practical strategies to identify, reduce, and manage indoor allergens in your home, you can create a healthier indoor environment and enjoy better respiratory health.

Controlling outdoor allergens: pollen, pollution, and weather changes

When it comes to managing asthma, outdoor allergens can pose significant challenges for individuals with asthma. Pollen, air pollution, and weather changes are among the most common outdoor triggers that can exacerbate asthma symptoms and lead to respiratory distress. In this chapter, we will explore practical strategies for identifying, minimizing exposure to, and managing these outdoor allergens to improve asthma control and respiratory health.

Pollen: Nature's Allergen

Pollen is a fine powder produced by plants, including trees, grasses, and weeds, as part of their reproductive process. When pollen becomes airborne, it can be inhaled by sensitive individuals and trigger allergic reactions, including asthma symptoms. Here's how to minimize exposure to pollen:

Monitor Pollen Counts: Stay informed about local pollen counts by checking weather reports or using pollen tracking apps. Limit outdoor activities on days when pollen levels are high, especially during peak pollen seasons.

Keep Windows Closed: Keep windows and doors closed during peak pollen seasons to prevent pollen from entering your home. Use air conditioning with a HEPA filter to filter out airborne pollen particles.

Shower and Change Clothes: After spending time outdoors, shower and change clothes to remove pollen from your hair and skin. This can help prevent pollen from being transferred to indoor surfaces.

Air Pollution: The Invisible Threat

Air pollution, including vehicle emissions, industrial pollutants, and particulate matter, can exacerbate asthma symptoms and decrease lung function in individuals with asthma. Minimizing exposure to air pollution is essential for maintaining respiratory health. Here's how to reduce exposure to air pollution:

Avoid Outdoor Exercise on High Pollution Days: Limit outdoor activities, especially strenuous exercise, on days when air pollution levels are high. Instead, opt for indoor exercise or activities in less polluted areas.

Use Air Purifiers: Consider using air purifiers with HEPA filters in your home to remove airborne pollutants and improve indoor air quality.

Choose Cleaner Transportation Options: Whenever possible, choose cleaner transportation options such as walking, biking, or using public transportation to reduce vehicle emissions and air pollution.

Weather Changes: The Asthma Agitator

Weather changes, including fluctuations in temperature, humidity, and barometric pressure, can trigger asthma symptoms in sensitive individuals. Cold air, high humidity, and sudden weather changes are common triggers for asthma exacerbations. Here's how to manage asthma symptoms during weather changes:

Dress Appropriately: Dress warmly in cold weather to protect your airways from the effects of cold air. Wear a scarf or mask over your nose and mouth to help warm and humidify the air you breathe.

Monitor Weather Forecasts: Stay informed about upcoming weather changes and plan accordingly. Take preventive measures, such as using asthma medications as prescribed, before anticipated weather changes occur.

Maintain Indoor Humidity Levels: Keep indoor humidity levels stable and within the optimal range (between 30%

and 50%) to minimize the impact of weather changes on asthma symptoms.

Lastly, controlling outdoor allergens such as pollen, air pollution, and weather changes is essential for individuals with asthma to reduce the frequency and severity of asthma symptoms and improve overall asthma control. By implementing practical strategies to minimize exposure to outdoor allergens and taking preventive measures during weather changes, you can effectively manage your asthma and enjoy better respiratory health.

CHAPTER FIVE

BREATHING TECHNIQUES FOR SUCCESS

5.1 LEARNING PROPER BREATHING EXERCISES AND TECHNIQUES

Mastering proper breathing exercises and techniques is essential for individuals with asthma to manage their symptoms, improve lung function, and enhance overall respiratory health. In this chapter, we will explore various breathing exercises and techniques that can help you breathe easier, reduce the frequency of asthma attacks, and enhance your quality of life.

Importance of Proper Breathing Techniques

Proper breathing techniques play a crucial role in asthma management by promoting optimal lung function, reducing respiratory muscle fatigue, and preventing hyperventilation. Learning to breathe effectively can help individuals with asthma maintain control over their symptoms and minimize the need for rescue medications. By incorporating breathing exercises into your daily routine, you can strengthen your respiratory muscles, improve oxygen exchange in the lungs, and reduce the sensation of breathlessness during physical activity.

Diaphragmatic Breathing: The Foundation of Healthy Breathing

Diaphragmatic breathing, also known as abdominal or belly breathing, involves engaging the diaphragm, the primary muscle responsible for breathing, to promote deeper and more efficient breathing. This technique helps to expand the lungs fully and allows for more oxygen to enter the body while facilitating the removal of carbon dioxide. To practice diaphragmatic breathing:

Find a Comfortable Position: Sit or lie down in a comfortable position with your back straight and shoulders relaxed.

Place One Hand on Your Chest and the Other on Your Abdomen: As you inhale slowly through your nose, focus on expanding your abdomen outward while keeping your chest relatively still

Exhale Slowly and Completely: Exhale slowly through pursed lips, allowing your abdomen to contract inward as you expel air from your lungs.

Repeat Several Times: Practice diaphragmatic breathing for several minutes each day, gradually increasing the duration and frequency as you become more comfortable with the technique.

Pursed-Lip Breathing: A Technique for Control

Pursed-lip breathing is a simple yet effective technique that can help individuals with asthma control their breathing during periods of breathlessness or exertion. This technique involves inhaling slowly through the nose and exhaling gently through pursed lips, creating a slight resistance to airflow that helps to prolong exhalation and prevent airway collapse. To practice pursed-lip breathing:

Inhale Slowly through Your Nose: Take a slow, deep breath in through your nose, focusing on filling your lungs completely.

Purse Your Lips: Pucker your lips as if you were going to whistle or blow out a candle.

Exhale Slowly and Gently: Exhale slowly and steadily through pursed lips, allowing the air to escape at a controlled pace. Aim to make your exhalation twice as long as your inhalation.

Relaxation Techniques for Managing Stress and Anxiety

Stress and anxiety can exacerbate asthma symptoms by triggering physiological responses such as shallow breathing and increased respiratory rate. Learning relaxation techniques can help individuals with asthma manage stress, reduce anxiety levels, and improve overall asthma control. Techniques such as progressive muscle relaxation, guided imagery, and deep breathing exercises can promote relaxation, alleviate muscle tension, and enhance feelings of calm and well-being.

Incorporating Breathing Exercises into Daily Life

To reap the benefits of breathing exercises, it's essential to incorporate them into your daily routine consistently. Practice diaphragmatic breathing, pursed-lip breathing, or relaxation techniques for a few minutes each day, ideally in a quiet and comfortable environment. You can integrate breathing exercises into activities such as yoga, meditation, or gentle stretching exercises to enhance their effectiveness and promote relaxation.

Mastering proper breathing exercises and techniques is a valuable skill for individuals with asthma to manage their symptoms, improve lung function, and enhance overall respiratory health. By incorporating diaphragmatic breathing, pursed-lip breathing, and relaxation techniques into your daily routine, you can strengthen your respiratory muscles, reduce stress and anxiety, and enjoy better asthma control. In the next chapter, we will delve into the importance of nutrition and exercise in asthma management and respiratory health.

5.2 Diaphragmatic breathing and pursed-lip breathing

In this section, we will explore two fundamental breathing techniques that can greatly benefit individuals with asthma: diaphragmatic breathing and pursed-lip breathing. These techniques are simple yet powerful tools for improving lung function, reducing breathlessness, and enhancing overall respiratory health.

Diaphragmatic Breathing: Harnessing the Power of the Diaphragm

Diaphragmatic breathing, also known as abdominal or belly breathing, involves engaging the diaphragm, the primary muscle responsible for breathing, to promote deeper and more efficient breathing. This technique facilitates optimal oxygen exchange in the lungs and helps to reduce the workload on accessory respiratory muscles, such as the neck and shoulders. By practicing diaphragmatic breathing regularly, individuals with asthma can enhance their lung capacity, improve ventilation-perfusion matching, and reduce the sensation of breathlessness during physical activity.

To practice diaphragmatic breathing:

Find a Quiet Space: Sit or lie down in a comfortable position in a quiet and relaxing environment.

Place One Hand on Your Chest and the Other on Your Abdomen: As you inhale slowly through your nose, focus on expanding your abdomen outward while keeping your chest relatively still.

Exhale Slowly and Completely: Exhale slowly through pursed lips, allowing your abdomen to contract inward as you expel air from your lungs.

Repeat Several Times: Practice diaphragmatic breathing for several minutes each day, gradually increasing the duration and frequency as you become more comfortable with the technique.

Pursed-Lip Breathing: Regulating Airflow for Control

Pursed-lip breathing is a breathing technique that involves inhaling slowly through the nose and exhaling gently through pursed lips. This technique creates a slight resistance to airflow during exhalation, prolonging the expiratory phase and preventing airway collapse. Pursed-lip breathing can help individuals with asthma control their breathing during periods of breathlessness or exertion, reduce the sensation of dyspnea, and improve overall asthma control.

To practice pursed-lip breathing:

Inhale Slowly through Your Nose: Take a slow, deep breath in through your nose, focusing on filling your lungs completely.

Purse Your Lips: Pucker your lips as if you were going to whistle or blow out a candle.

Exhale Slowly and Gently: Exhale slowly and steadily through pursed lips, allowing the air to escape at a controlled pace. Aim to make your exhalation twice as long as your inhalation.

Incorporating Breathing Techniques into Daily Life

Both diaphragmatic breathing and pursed-lip breathing can be easily integrated into daily life and incorporated into various activities to enhance their effectiveness. Individuals with asthma can practice these techniques during rest periods, before and after physical activity, or when experiencing asthma symptoms such as breathlessness or chest tightness. Consistent practice of these breathing techniques can help individuals with asthma improve their lung function, reduce stress and anxiety, and enhance overall respiratory health.

Diaphragmatic breathing and pursed-lip breathing are two valuable tools for individuals with asthma to improve lung function, reduce breathlessness, and enhance overall respiratory health. By incorporating these simple yet effective breathing techniques into their daily routine, individuals with asthma can strengthen their respiratory muscles, improve oxygen exchange in the lungs, and enjoy better asthma control.

5.3 Relaxation techniques for managing stress and anxiety

In the fast-paced world we live in, stress and anxiety have become increasingly prevalent, affecting individuals of all ages and backgrounds. For individuals with asthma, stress and anxiety can exacerbate symptoms, trigger asthma attacks, and impact overall respiratory health. In this chapter, we will explore various relaxation techniques that can help individuals with asthma manage stress, reduce anxiety levels, and improve asthma control.

The Impact of Stress and Anxiety on Asthma

Stress and anxiety can have a significant impact on asthma symptoms and overall respiratory health. When we experience stress or anxiety, our body's natural response is to release stress hormones such as cortisol and adrenaline, which can trigger physiological changes in the body, including shallow breathing, increased heart rate, and muscle tension. These changes can exacerbate asthma symptoms, leading to airway inflammation, bronchoconstriction, and respiratory distress. By learning to manage stress and anxiety effectively, individuals with asthma can reduce the frequency and severity of asthma attacks and improve overall asthma control.

Progressive Muscle Relaxation: Unwinding Body and Mind

Progressive muscle relaxation is a relaxation technique that involves tensing and then relaxing different muscle groups in the body to promote deep relaxation and reduce muscle tension. This technique helps individuals with asthma release physical tension, alleviate muscle stiffness, and induce a state of calm and relaxation. To practice progressive muscle relaxation:

Find a Quiet Space: Sit or lie down in a comfortable position in a quiet and peaceful environment.

Progressive Muscle Tension: Start by tensing the muscles in your toes and feet, holding the tension for a few seconds, and then releasing the tension completely. Gradually work your way up the body, tensing and relaxing each muscle group, including the legs, abdomen, chest, arms, shoulders, and face.

Deep Breathing: As you tense and relax each muscle group, focus on your breath. Inhale slowly and deeply through your nose as you tense the muscles, and exhale slowly and completely through your mouth as you release the tension.

Guided Imagery: Harnessing the Power of Visualization

Guided imagery is a relaxation technique that involves using visualization to create mental images that evoke a sense of calm and well-being. By immersing oneself in a peaceful and tranquil imaginary scene, individuals with asthma can reduce stress and anxiety levels, promote relaxation, and enhance overall respiratory health. To practice guided imagery:

Choose a Peaceful Scene: Close your eyes and visualize yourself in a peaceful and serene location, such as a beach, forest, or mountainside.

Engage Your Senses: Engage all your senses in the visualization process. Imagine the sights, sounds, smells, textures, and tastes of your chosen scene in vivid detail.

Focus on Relaxation: As you immerse yourself in the imaginary scene, focus on relaxing your body and mind. Take slow, deep breaths and allow yourself to let go of any tension or stress you may be holding onto.

Deep Breathing Exercises: Calming the Mind and Body

Deep breathing exercises, such as diaphragmatic breathing and pursed-lip breathing, are powerful tools for promoting relaxation, reducing stress and anxiety, and improving overall respiratory health. By focusing on slow, deep breaths and engaging the diaphragm, individuals with asthma can activate the body's natural relaxation response, lower stress hormone levels, and enhance feelings of calm and well-being.

In conclusion, Relaxation techniques are valuable tools for individuals with asthma to manage stress, reduce anxiety levels, and improve overall asthma control. By incorporating progressive muscle relaxation, guided imagery, deep breathing exercises, and other relaxation techniques into their daily routine, individuals with asthma can promote relaxation, alleviate muscle tension, and enhance respiratory health.

CHAPTER SIX

NUTRITION AND EXERCISE

6.1 UNDERSTANDING THE LINK BETWEEN DIET AND ASTHMA

Diet plays a significant role in overall health and well-being, and emerging research suggests that it may also influence asthma symptoms and respiratory health. In this chapter, we will explore the complex relationship between diet and asthma, examining how dietary factors can impact asthma risk, symptom severity, and disease management.

The Role of Inflammation in Asthma

Inflammation is a key component of asthma, contributing to airway hyperresponsiveness, bronchoconstriction, and respiratory symptoms. Certain dietary factors have been found to modulate inflammation in the body, potentially influencing asthma outcomes. Understanding the impact of diet on inflammation can provide valuable insights into asthma management and treatment.

Anti-Inflammatory Foods: Nourishing Your Body

Some foods possess anti-inflammatory properties and may help to reduce inflammation in the body. These foods are rich in antioxidants, vitamins, minerals, and phytochemicals that have been shown to combat inflammation and support overall health. Incorporating anti-inflammatory foods into your diet may help to alleviate asthma symptoms and improve respiratory function. Examples of anti-inflammatory foods include:

Fatty Fish: Rich in omega-3 fatty acids, fatty fish such as salmon, mackerel, and sardines have potent anti-inflammatory effects and may help to reduce airway inflammation in individuals with asthma.

Fruits and Vegetables: Colorful fruits and vegetables are packed with antioxidants, vitamins, and phytochemicals that can help to reduce inflammation and support respiratory health. Aim to include a variety of fruits and vegetables in your diet, such as berries, leafy greens, bell peppers, and tomatoes.

Nuts and Seeds: Nuts and seeds are excellent sources of healthy fats, fiber, and antioxidants that can help to reduce inflammation and improve asthma control. Incorporate nuts and seeds such as almonds, walnuts, flaxseeds, and chia seeds into your meals and snacks.

Whole Grains: Whole grains such as oats, quinoa, brown rice, and barley are rich in fiber and nutrients that can help to regulate inflammation and support respiratory health. Choose whole grains over refined grains to maximize their anti-inflammatory benefits.

Trigger Foods: Identifying Potential Culprits

While some foods may help to reduce inflammation and support respiratory health, others may trigger or exacerbate asthma symptoms in susceptible individuals. These trigger foods vary from person to person and may include common allergens, food additives, and preservatives. Identifying and avoiding trigger foods can help to minimize asthma symptoms and improve overall asthma control. Common trigger foods for individuals with asthma may include:

Dairy Products: Some individuals with asthma may be sensitive to dairy products such as milk, cheese, and yogurt, which can trigger mucus production and airway inflammation.

Sulfites: Sulfites are commonly used as preservatives in processed foods and beverages and may trigger asthma symptoms in sensitive individuals. Avoiding foods and drinks containing sulfites can help to prevent asthma exacerbations.

Processed Foods: Processed foods high in sugar, refined carbohydrates, and unhealthy fats may promote inflammation in the body and exacerbate asthma symptoms. opt for whole, unprocessed foods whenever possible to support respiratory health.

The Gut Microbiome: A Key Player in Asthma

Emerging research suggests that the gut microbiome, the community of microorganisms that inhabit the digestive tract, may play a crucial role in asthma development and progression. The composition and diversity of the gut microbiome can influence immune function, inflammation, and respiratory health. Certain dietary factors, such as fiber-rich foods and probiotics, may help to promote a healthy gut microbiome and reduce asthma risk.

The link between diet and asthma is complex and multifaceted, with dietary factors playing a significant role in asthma risk, symptom severity, and disease management. By incorporating anti-inflammatory foods, identifying and avoiding trigger foods, and promoting a healthy gut microbiome, individuals with asthma can optimize their diet to support respiratory health and improve asthma control.

6.2 Choosing healthy foods and avoiding inflammatory triggers

In the quest for optimal health and well-being, the role of nutrition cannot be overstated. When it comes to managing asthma, making informed choices about the foods we eat can have a significant impact on symptom control and overall respiratory health. In this chapter, we will explore the principles of choosing healthy foods while avoiding inflammatory triggers to support asthma management and enhance quality of life.

Understanding Inflammatory Triggers

Inflammation lies at the heart of asthma, contributing to airway constriction, mucus production, and respiratory symptoms. Certain dietary factors have been identified as potential triggers for inflammation in the body, exacerbating asthma symptoms and compromising respiratory health. By recognizing these inflammatory triggers and making conscious decisions to avoid them, individuals with asthma can better manage their condition and improve asthma control.

Common Inflammatory Triggers to Avoid

Processed Foods: Processed foods, including sugary snacks, refined grains, and packaged meals, are often high in unhealthy fats, sugars, and additives that can promote inflammation in the body. To reduce inflammation and support respiratory health, opt for whole, unprocessed foods whenever possible.

Trans Fats: Trans fats are artificial fats found in fried foods, baked goods, and processed snacks. These fats can increase levels of inflammatory markers in the body and exacerbate asthma symptoms. Choose foods rich in healthy fats, such as avocados, nuts, seeds, and olive oil, instead of trans fats.

High-Sugar Foods: Diets high in sugar have been linked to increased inflammation and oxidative stress in the body, which can worsen asthma symptoms and impair respiratory function. Minimize your intake of sugary foods and beverages, such as soda, candy, and sweetened snacks, to support respiratory health.

Embracing Anti-Inflammatory Foods

In contrast to inflammatory triggers, certain foods possess anti-inflammatory properties and can help to reduce inflammation in the body. These foods are rich in antioxidants, vitamins, minerals, and phytochemicals that have been shown to combat inflammation and support overall health. By incorporating anti-inflammatory foods into your diet, you can promote respiratory health and improve asthma control.

Anti-Inflammatory Foods to Include

Fruits and Vegetables: Colorful fruits and vegetables are rich in antioxidants, vitamins, and phytochemicals that can help to reduce inflammation and support respiratory health. Aim to include a variety of fruits and vegetables in your diet, such as berries, leafy greens, citrus fruits, and cruciferous vegetables.

Fatty Fish: Fatty fish such as salmon, mackerel, and trout are excellent sources of omega-3 fatty acids, which have potent anti-inflammatory effects. Incorporating fatty fish into your diet regularly can help to reduce airway inflammation and improve asthma control.

Whole Grains: Whole grains such as oats, quinoa, brown rice, and barley are rich in fiber and nutrients that can help to regulate inflammation and support respiratory health.

Choose whole grains over refined grains to maximize their anti-inflammatory benefits.

Choosing healthy foods while avoiding inflammatory triggers is essential for individuals with asthma to support respiratory health and improve asthma control. By recognizing common inflammatory triggers and embracing anti-inflammatory foods, individuals with asthma can optimize their diet to reduce inflammation, alleviate symptoms, and enhance overall well-being.

6.3 Incorporating safe and effective exercise into your routine

Exercise is a cornerstone of a healthy lifestyle, offering numerous benefits for both physical and mental well-being. For individuals with asthma, incorporating exercise into their routine can be particularly beneficial, helping to improve lung function, enhance respiratory muscle strength, and reduce asthma symptoms. In this chapter, we will explore practical strategies for safely and effectively integrating exercise into your daily life, allowing you to reap the rewards of physical activity while managing your asthma effectively.

Understanding Exercise-Induced Asthma

Exercise-induced asthma, also known as exercise-induced bronchoconstriction, is a common condition characterized by the narrowing of the airways during or after physical activity. For individuals with asthma, exercise can trigger symptoms such as coughing, wheezing, chest tightness, and shortness of breath. However, with proper management and precautions, individuals with asthma can participate in regular exercise and enjoy its many benefits.

Choosing the Right Types of Exercise

When it comes to exercising with asthma, not all activities are created equal. Certain types of exercise may be more asthma-friendly than others, minimizing the risk of triggering symptoms and promoting respiratory health. Low-impact activities that involve continuous, rhythmic movements, such as walking, cycling, swimming, and yoga, are generally well-tolerated by individuals with asthma. These activities help to improve cardiovascular fitness, strengthen respiratory muscles, and enhance lung function without placing excessive strain on the airways.

Pre-Exercise Preparation

Before engaging in physical activity, individuals with asthma should take steps to prepare their bodies and minimize the risk of asthma symptoms. This may include:

Pre-Exercise Medication: Taking prescribed asthma medications, such as bronchodilators or controller medications, as directed by your healthcare provider before exercise can help to prevent exercise-induced symptoms and improve exercise tolerance.

Warm-Up: Performing a gentle warm-up routine before exercise can help to gradually increase heart rate, improve blood flow to the muscles, and prepare the respiratory system for physical activity. Incorporating dynamic stretches, light aerobic exercises, and breathing exercises into your warm-up routine can help to reduce the risk of asthma symptoms during exercise.

Hydration: Staying hydrated is essential for individuals with asthma, particularly during exercise. Drinking water before, during, and after physical activity can help to keep the airways moist and prevent dehydration, which can exacerbate asthma symptoms.

Monitoring Symptoms During Exercise

During exercise, it is important for individuals with asthma to pay attention to their bodies and monitor for any signs of asthma symptoms. If you experience symptoms such as coughing, wheezing, chest tightness, or shortness of breath, it is essential to take appropriate action to manage your asthma and prevent symptom escalation. This may include:

Stopping Exercise: If you experience asthma symptoms during exercise, stop physical activity immediately and rest until symptoms subside. Use your prescribed rescue inhaler as directed by your healthcare provider to relieve symptoms and open up the airways.

Seeking Medical Attention: If asthma symptoms persist or worsen despite using your rescue inhaler, seek medical attention promptly. Your healthcare provider can assess your symptoms, adjust your asthma treatment plan if necessary, and provide guidance on safely resuming physical activity.

Gradual Progression and Consistency

When incorporating exercise into your routine, it is important to start slowly and gradually increase the intensity and duration of physical activity over time. This allows your body to adapt to the demands of exercise and reduces the risk of triggering asthma symptoms. Consistency is key when it comes to reaping the benefits of exercise for asthma management. Aim to engage in regular physical activity on most days of the week, incorporating a mix of aerobic, strength training, and flexibility exercises to promote overall health and respiratory function.

Incorporating safe and effective exercise into your routine is an important component of asthma management, offering numerous benefits for respiratory health and overall well-being. By choosing asthma-friendly activities, taking appropriate precautions, monitoring symptoms during exercise, and gradually progressing your fitness level, you can enjoy the rewards of physical activity while effectively managing your asthma.

6.4 Modifying exercise plans for different asthma severities

When it comes to managing asthma through exercise, it's crucial to recognize that the severity of asthma symptoms can vary greatly from person to person. What works well for one individual may not be suitable for another, depending on factors such as asthma severity, triggers, and overall health. In this chapter, we will explore strategies for modifying exercise plans to accommodate different asthma severities, ensuring that individuals with asthma can safely and effectively incorporate physical activity into their lives.

Understanding Asthma Severity

Asthma severity refers to the intensity and frequency of asthma symptoms, as well as the degree of airflow limitation and respiratory impairment. Asthma severity can range from mild intermittent asthma, characterized by infrequent and mild symptoms, to severe persistent asthma, marked by frequent and severe symptoms that significantly impact daily life. Understanding your asthma severity is essential for tailoring your exercise plan to meet your individual needs and capabilities.

Modifying Exercise Intensity and Duration

For individuals with mild intermittent asthma, exercise plans can typically be more flexible, with fewer limitations on intensity and duration. However, it's still important to listen to your body and avoid pushing yourself too hard, particularly if you experience asthma symptoms during physical activity. Taking regular breaks, pacing yourself, and monitoring your symptoms closely can help to prevent symptom exacerbation and ensure a safe and enjoyable exercise experience.

For individuals with moderate to severe asthma, it may be necessary to modify exercise intensity and duration more significantly to accommodate respiratory limitations and reduce the risk of symptom exacerbation. This may involve:

Choosing Low-Impact Activities: Opting for low-impact exercises such as walking, cycling, swimming, or yoga can help to minimize the strain on the airways and reduce the risk of triggering asthma symptoms.

Shorter, More Frequent Sessions: Breaking up your exercise routine into shorter, more frequent sessions throughout the day can help to reduce the overall intensity and duration of physical activity while still reaping the benefits of exercise.

Gradual Progression: Gradually increasing the intensity and duration of physical activity over time, rather than pushing yourself too hard too soon, can help to build endurance and improve fitness while minimizing the risk of asthma symptoms.

Special Considerations for Severe Asthma

For individuals with severe persistent asthma, managing exercise can pose unique challenges due to the severity of symptoms and the potential for frequent exacerbations. In these cases, it's essential to work closely with your healthcare provider to develop a personalized exercise plan that takes into account your specific needs and limitations. Your healthcare provider may recommend additional precautions, such as:

Pre-Exercise Medication: Taking prescribed asthma medications, such as bronchodilators or controller medications, before exercise can help to prevent exercise-induced symptoms and improve exercise tolerance.

Close Monitoring: Monitoring your symptoms closely during and after exercise and adjusting your activity level accordingly can help to prevent symptom exacerbation and ensure your safety.

Modifying exercise plans for different asthma severities is essential for ensuring that individuals with asthma can safely and effectively incorporate physical activity into their lives. By understanding your asthma severity, choosing appropriate activities, modifying exercise intensity and duration as needed, and working closely with your healthcare provider, you can enjoy the benefits of exercise while effectively managing your asthma.

CHAPTER SEVEN

EMOTIONAL WELLBEING AND ASTHMA

7.1 THE IMPACT OF ASTHMA ON MENTAL HEALTH AND VICE VERSA

Living with asthma can be challenging, not only due to the physical symptoms and limitations it imposes but also because of its impact on mental health. In this chapter, we will explore the complex interplay between asthma and mental health, examining how asthma can affect psychological well-being and vice versa.

The Psychological Burden of Asthma

For many individuals with asthma, the constant threat of asthma attacks, the need for ongoing medication, and the limitations on daily activities can take a toll on mental health. Anxiety, depression, and stress are common psychological responses to living with a chronic condition like asthma. The fear of experiencing an asthma attack or not being able to breathe properly can lead to heightened anxiety levels, which may exacerbate asthma symptoms in a vicious cycle.

Managing Asthma-related Anxiety and Stress

Coping with asthma-related anxiety and stress requires a multifaceted approach that addresses both the physical and psychological aspects of the condition. Strategies for managing asthma-related anxiety and stress may include:

Education and Self-Management: Learning more about asthma, its triggers, and how to effectively manage symptoms can empower individuals with asthma and help to reduce anxiety and stress.

Relaxation Techniques: Practicing relaxation techniques such as deep breathing, meditation, and progressive muscle relaxation can help to calm the mind and reduce stress levels.

Cognitive-Behavioral Therapy (CBT): CBT is a type of psychotherapy that focuses on identifying and challenging negative thought patterns and developing coping skills to manage anxiety and stress.

Support Networks: Seeking support from friends, family members, support groups, or mental health professionals can provide valuable emotional support and practical coping strategies for managing asthma-related anxiety and stress.

The Bidirectional Relationship between Asthma and Mental Health

While asthma can have a significant impact on mental health, the relationship between asthma and mental health is bidirectional, meaning that mental health issues can also influence asthma outcomes. Research suggests that individuals with pre-existing mental health conditions such as anxiety and depression may be at increased risk of asthma exacerbations and poorer asthma control.

Addressing Mental Health in Asthma Management

Given the bidirectional relationship between asthma and mental health, addressing mental health issues is an important aspect of asthma management. Healthcare providers should routinely assess the psychological well-being of individuals with asthma and provide appropriate support and resources as needed. This may include referrals to mental health professionals, counseling services, or support groups.

The impact of asthma on mental health and vice versa is a complex and multifaceted issue that requires careful attention and consideration. By addressing the psychological aspects of asthma and incorporating strategies to manage asthma-related anxiety and stress, individuals with asthma can improve their overall quality of life and asthma outcomes.

7.2 Managing stress, anxiety, and depression

Living with asthma can be overwhelming at times, especially when faced with the challenges of managing symptoms, avoiding triggers, and navigating daily life. Stress, anxiety, and depression are common emotional responses to living with a chronic condition like asthma, but they don't have to define your experience.

Recognizing the Signs and Symptoms

Stress, anxiety, and depression can manifest in a variety of ways, both emotionally and physically. Common signs and symptoms may include feelings of worry or unease, difficulty concentrating, changes in appetite or sleep patterns, fatigue, irritability, and physical symptoms such as muscle tension or headaches. Recognizing these signs and acknowledging their impact on your well-being is the first step toward effective management.

Developing Coping Strategies

Coping with stress, anxiety, and depression requires a proactive approach that incorporates a variety of coping strategies tailored to your individual needs. Some effective coping strategies may include:

Mindfulness and Relaxation Techniques: Practicing mindfulness, deep breathing exercises, meditation, or progressive muscle relaxation can help to calm the mind and reduce stress and anxiety levels.

Physical Activity: Engaging in regular physical activity, such as walking, cycling, or yoga, can help to improve mood, reduce stress, and promote overall well-being.

Social Support: Seeking support from friends, family members, support groups, or mental health professionals can provide valuable emotional support and practical coping strategies.

Healthy Lifestyle Habits: Prioritizing self-care activities such as getting enough sleep, eating a balanced diet, and avoiding excessive alcohol or caffeine consumption can help to support overall mental and emotional well-being.

Seeking Professional Help

In some cases, managing stress, anxiety, and depression may require professional intervention. If you find that your symptoms are significantly impacting your daily life or functioning, it's important to seek help from a qualified mental health professional. Therapy, counseling, or medication may be recommended as part of a comprehensive treatment plan to address underlying issues and provide effective symptom relief.

Integrating Mental Health into Asthma Management

Recognizing the interconnectedness of mental and physical health is essential for effective asthma management. Integrating mental health into your asthma management plan can help to improve overall well-being and asthma outcomes. Healthcare providers should routinely assess the psychological well-being of individuals with asthma and provide appropriate support and resources as needed.

Managing stress, anxiety, and depression while living with asthma is a journey that requires patience, self-awareness, and resilience. By recognizing the signs and symptoms, developing effective coping strategies, seeking support when needed, and integrating mental health into asthma management, individuals with asthma can improve their overall quality of life and well-being.

7.3 Building resilience and a positive outlook

Living with asthma can sometimes feel like an uphill battle, but building resilience and maintaining a positive outlook are key to managing the condition effectively and leading a fulfilling life. This chapter explores strategies for fostering resilience and cultivating a positive mindset, which are essential for overcoming challenges and thriving despite asthma.

Understanding Resilience

Resilience is the ability to adapt and bounce back from adversity. It's about-facing challenges head-on, learning from experiences, and emerging stronger. For those living with asthma, resilience involves managing symptoms, coping with setbacks, and maintaining a sense of control and optimism.

Strategies for Building Resilience

Set Realistic Goals: Setting achievable, short-term goals can provide a sense of purpose and direction. Whether it's improving your asthma management, increasing your physical activity, or developing a new skill, having goals to work towards can be motivating and rewarding.

Develop a Support Network: Surround yourself with supportive friends, family, and healthcare providers who understand your condition and can offer encouragement and assistance. Connecting with others who have asthma can also provide valuable insights and a sense of community.

Practice Self-Care: Taking care of your physical and mental health is crucial for building resilience. This includes regular exercise, a balanced diet, sufficient sleep, and engaging in activities that you enjoy and find relaxing.

Learn from Experiences: Reflect on past experiences with asthma to identify what strategies have worked well and what could be improved. Use these insights to make informed decisions about your asthma management.

Maintain a Routine: Establishing a daily routine can provide structure and predictability, which can be comforting during times of stress. Include regular medication, monitoring, and relaxation practices in your routine to stay on top of your asthma management.

Stay Informed: Educate yourself about asthma and stay updated on the latest treatments and management strategies. Knowledge is empowering and can help you feel more in control of your condition.

Cultivating a Positive Outlook

Focus on What You Can Control: While you can't control having asthma, you can control how you manage it. Focus on the actions you can take to improve your health and well-being rather than the limitations imposed by the condition.

Practice Gratitude: Regularly take time to reflect on the positive aspects of your life. Keeping a gratitude journal or sharing positive experiences with others can help shift your focus from challenges to blessings.

Embrace Positive Thinking: Challenge negative thoughts and replace them with positive affirmations. Remind yourself of your strengths, achievements, and the progress you've made in managing your asthma.

Stay Engaged in Life: Pursue hobbies, interests, and activities that bring you joy and fulfillment. Staying engaged in meaningful activities can provide a sense of purpose and help maintain a positive outlook.

Seek Professional Help When Needed: If you're struggling to maintain a positive outlook or find that stress, anxiety, or depression are affecting your quality of life, seek help from a mental health professional. Therapy and counseling can provide valuable tools and support for managing emotional challenges.

The Power of Resilience and Positivity

Building resilience and maintaining a positive outlook are powerful tools in managing asthma. They enable you to face challenges with confidence, adapt to changes, and continue to pursue your goals and dreams. Remember, resilience is not about being invulnerable; it's about recognizing your capacity to recover and grow stronger from adversity.

Living with asthma requires a proactive and resilient approach. By setting realistic goals, developing a support network, practicing self-care, and cultivating a positive outlook, you can navigate the challenges of asthma with grace and determination.

CHAPTER EIGHT

SCHOOL, WORK, AND PLAY

ADVOCATING FOR YOURSELF AND YOUR NEEDS IN DIFFERENT SETTINGS

Living with asthma means that you'll need to be proactive in managing your condition across various aspects of your life. Advocating for yourself—whether at school, work, or social settings—is crucial to ensuring you get the support and accommodations you need. This chapter will guide you through the strategies to effectively communicate your needs and take charge of your asthma management in different environments.

Understanding Self-Advocacy

Self-advocacy involves speaking up for yourself, understanding your rights, and making informed decisions about your health. It means taking responsibility for your well-being and ensuring that others understand and respect your needs.

Advocating for Yourself at School

Informing School Staff: Communicate with teachers, school nurses, and administrators about your asthma. Provide them with a detailed asthma action plan, which outlines your triggers, symptoms, medications, and emergency procedures.

Creating a Safe Environment: Work with school staff to minimize exposure to common asthma triggers such as dust, mold, and strong odors. Ensure that your classroom and other areas are well-ventilated and clean.

Managing Physical Activity: Discuss your limitations and needs regarding physical activities with your physical education teacher. Ensure that you have access to your rescue inhaler during exercise and that alternative activities are available if needed.

Educating Peers: Educating your classmates about asthma can foster understanding and support. Consider giving a short presentation or providing informational materials to raise awareness about your condition.

Advocating for Yourself at Work

Disclosing Your Condition: Deciding whether to disclose your asthma at work is a personal choice. If you choose to disclose, provide your employer and colleagues with the necessary information about your condition and how they can support you.

Requesting Accommodations: The Americans with Disabilities Act (ADA) requires employers to provide reasonable accommodations for employees with chronic conditions. This could include modifying your workspace, allowing flexible break times for medication, or providing an air purifier.

Creating an Asthma-Friendly Workspace: Work with your employer to ensure that your workspace is free from common asthma triggers such as smoke, strong odors, and allergens. Regular cleaning and good ventilation are essential.

Managing Stress: Work-related stress can exacerbate asthma symptoms. Practice stress management techniques such as deep breathing, mindfulness, and regular breaks to help maintain your well-being.

Advocating for Yourself in Social Settings

Communicating with Friends and Family: Educate your friends and family about your asthma, including your triggers, symptoms, and emergency procedures. This will help them understand your condition and provide the necessary support.

Planning Ahead: When attending social events, plan ahead to ensure that your needs are met. This might involve bringing your medication, identifying a quiet space for breaks, or informing the host about your condition.

Managing Environmental Triggers: Be mindful of potential triggers in social settings, such as smoke, strong fragrances, and pets. Don't hesitate to politely request that these triggers be minimized or avoided.

Practicing Assertiveness: Practice being assertive when communicating your needs. Use clear and direct language, and don't be afraid to stand up for yourself if you feel your needs are not being respected.

Advocating for Yourself in Healthcare Settings

Building a Relationship with Your Healthcare Team: Establish open and honest communication with your healthcare providers. Share your concerns, ask questions, and ensure that you understand your treatment plan.

Preparing for Appointments: Write down your symptoms, questions, and any changes in your condition before your appointments. This will help you make the most of your time with your healthcare provider.

Seeking Second Opinions: If you feel that your concerns are not being addressed or your treatment is not effective, don't hesitate to seek a second opinion. It's important to find a healthcare provider who listens to you and respects your needs.

Understanding Your Rights: Familiarize yourself with your rights as a patient. You have the right to receive clear information, participate in decisions about your care, and refuse or accept treatment.

The Power of Self-Advocacy

Advocating for yourself empowers you to take control of your asthma management and improve your quality of life. It helps ensure that your environment is safe and supportive, allowing you to focus on your goals and activities without the constant worry of asthma flare-ups.

8.2 Managing asthma at school and work

Asthma can present unique challenges in both school and work environments, but with the right strategies and support, you can effectively manage your condition and excel in these settings. This chapter offers practical advice on navigating the complexities of asthma management at school and work, ensuring you stay healthy and productive.

Strategies for Managing Asthma at School

1. Communication with School Staff:

One of the most critical steps in managing asthma at school is establishing open communication with teachers, school nurses, and administrators. Inform them about your child's asthma, provide an updated asthma action plan, and ensure they understand how to respond in case of an emergency.

2. Individualized Health Plans:

Request an Individualized Health Plan (IHP) for your child. This plan should outline specific asthma management strategies, including medication schedules, trigger avoidance, and emergency procedures. For students with severe asthma, a 504 Plan or Individualized Education Program (IEP) can provide additional accommodations.

3. Medication Management:

Ensure that your child has easy access to their asthma medications during school hours. Work with the school nurse to store and administer medications if necessary. It's essential that your child knows how to use their inhaler correctly and understands the importance of taking their medications as prescribed.

4. Reducing Exposure to Triggers:

Identify potential asthma triggers within the school environment and work with school staff to minimize exposure. Common triggers include dust, mold, pet dander, and strong odors. Advocate for regular cleaning, proper ventilation, and allergen-free classrooms.

5. Physical Activity:

Physical activity is crucial for overall health but can be challenging for students with asthma. Ensure that your child's PE teacher is aware of their condition and understands how to manage it during physical activities. Allow your child to use their rescue inhaler before exercise and provide alternatives if needed.

6. Education and Awareness:

Educating classmates and teachers about asthma can create a more supportive and understanding environment. Consider giving a brief presentation or distributing informational materials to raise awareness about asthma and its management.

7. Emergency Preparedness:

Ensure that all school staff are trained to recognize asthma symptoms and respond appropriately during an asthma attack. The asthma action plan should be easily accessible, and everyone should know the location of emergency medications.

Strategies for Managing Asthma at Work

1. Disclosure and Communication:

Deciding whether to disclose your asthma at work is a personal decision. If you choose to disclose, communicate your needs clearly to your employer and colleagues. Provide them with information about your condition, triggers, and what to do in an emergency.

2. Requesting Accommodations:

Under the Americans with Disabilities Act (ADA), you have the right to request reasonable accommodations to help manage your asthma at work. This could include adjustments to your workspace, such as improved ventilation, a smoke-free environment, or the use of air purifiers.

3. Medication Accessibility:

Keep your asthma medications, including rescue inhalers, easily accessible during work hours. Make sure you have a plan for taking your medications as needed and inform your employer if you might need to take breaks to manage your asthma.

4. Reducing Workplace Triggers:

Identify and address potential asthma triggers in your workplace. Common triggers include dust, strong odors, chemical fumes, and poor air quality. Work with your employer to mitigate these triggers, which might involve changing cleaning products, improving ventilation, or relocating your workspace.

5. Managing Stress:

Work-related stress can exacerbate asthma symptoms. Practice stress management techniques such as deep breathing, mindfulness, and regular breaks. Consider setting realistic goals and prioritizing tasks to manage your workload effectively.

6. Healthy Lifestyle Choices:

Maintaining a healthy lifestyle can help manage asthma symptoms. Eat a balanced diet, exercise regularly, and get enough sleep. Staying hydrated and avoiding smoking or exposure to secondhand smoke are also important.

7. Emergency Preparedness:

Ensure that your colleagues are aware of your asthma and know how to respond in an emergency. Keep your asthma action plan accessible and review it with your supervisor and HR department. Conduct regular drills if necessary to ensure everyone is prepared.

Balancing School, Work, and Asthma Management

Balancing asthma management with the demands of school or work can be challenging, but it's essential for your overall well-being. Here are some additional tips to help you succeed

1. Time Management:

Effective time management can reduce stress and help you stay on top of your asthma management. Plan your day, set priorities, and allow time for rest and medication.

2. Support Networks:

Build a support network of friends, family, and colleagues who understand your condition and can provide assistance when needed. Joining an asthma support group can also be beneficial for sharing experiences and advice.

3. Regular Check-ups:

Keep regular appointments with your healthcare provider to monitor your asthma and adjust your treatment plan as needed. Inform your doctor about any changes in your school or work environment that might affect your asthma.

4. Staying Informed:

Stay informed about asthma and its management by reading reputable sources, attending workshops, and participating in online forums. Knowledge empowers you to make informed decisions about your health.

5. Self-Care:

Prioritize self-care and listen to your body. Take breaks when needed, practice relaxation techniques, and don't hesitate to seek help if you're feeling overwhelmed.

Managing asthma at school and work requires proactive planning, effective communication, and a supportive environment. By advocating for yourself, staying informed, and implementing these strategies, you can successfully manage your asthma and achieve your goals.

8.3 Participating in sports and activities with asthma

Asthma doesn't have to limit your ability to participate in sports and physical activities. In fact, staying active is beneficial for overall health and can improve asthma management. With proper planning, understanding your body's signals, and following a few key strategies, you can enjoy and excel in various sports and activities. This chapter will guide you through the essentials of staying active while managing asthma effectively.

Benefits of Physical Activity for People with Asthma

Engaging in regular physical activity offers numerous benefits for people with asthma:

Improved Lung Function: Regular exercise helps strengthen the respiratory muscles, improving lung function and breathing efficiency.

Enhanced Immune System: Physical activity boosts the immune system, reducing the frequency of respiratory infections that can trigger asthma.

Better Weight Management: Maintaining a healthy weight can alleviate asthma symptoms and reduce the burden on the respiratory system.

Stress Reduction: Exercise is a great way to manage stress, which can be a common asthma trigger.

Overall Fitness: Staying active improves overall cardiovascular fitness, endurance, and energy levels.

Choosing the Right Activities

While most sports and physical activities can be safe for people with asthma, some are more asthma-friendly than others. Here are a few considerations:

Low to Moderate Intensity Activities:

Walking, swimming, biking, and yoga are generally well-tolerated by people with asthma. These activities are less likely to provoke asthma symptoms compared to high-intensity or endurance sports.

Warm-Up and Cool-Down:

Always include a proper warm-up and cool-down routine. Gradually increasing your heart rate before exercise and slowly bringing it down afterward can help prevent asthma symptoms.

Swimming:

Swimming is often recommended for people with asthma because the warm, humid air of the pool environment is less likely to trigger symptoms. It's also a great full-body workout.

Team Sports:

Sports like baseball, volleyball, and tennis involve short bursts of activity and rest periods, making them suitable for people with asthma. Ensure to communicate with teammates and coaches about your condition.

Preparing for Physical Activity

Proper preparation is key to managing asthma during physical activity:

Asthma Action Plan:

Have an up-to-date asthma action plan developed with your healthcare provider. This plan should outline what to do before, during, and after exercise, including when to use medication.

Medication Management:

Use your prescribed inhaler or medication as directed by your doctor. This might include using a short-acting bronchodilator (rescue inhaler) 15-20 minutes before starting exercise.

Monitor Your Condition:

Keep track of your asthma symptoms and peak flow readings. This helps you understand how your body responds to different activities and environments.

Hydration:

Stay well-hydrated before, during, and after exercise. Dehydration can exacerbate asthma symptoms.

Avoid Triggers:

Be aware of and avoid potential asthma triggers such as pollen, cold air, pollution, and strong odors. If exercising outdoors, check the air quality and pollen levels beforehand.

Managing Symptoms During Exercise

Knowing how to manage symptoms that arise during exercise can help you stay active safely:

Recognize Early Symptoms:

Learn to recognize early signs of asthma, such as coughing, wheezing, chest tightness, or shortness of breath. Stop the activity if these symptoms occur.

Use Rescue Inhaler:

If symptoms develop, use your rescue inhaler as directed. Wait for the medication to take effect before resuming activity.

Pace Yourself:

Gradually increase the intensity and duration of your workouts. Listen to your body and take breaks as needed.

Breathe Through Your Nose:

Breathing through your nose can help warm and humidify the air before it reaches your lungs, reducing the likelihood of triggering asthma symptoms.

Long-Term Strategies for Active Living

To maintain an active lifestyle with asthma, consider the following long-term strategies:

Regular Check-Ups:

Schedule regular check-ups with your healthcare provider to monitor your asthma and adjust your treatment plan as needed.

Asthma Education:

Stay informed about asthma management through reliable sources. Understanding your condition empowers you to make better decisions about your health and activity levels.

Support System:

Build a support network of family, friends, coaches, and healthcare providers who understand your condition and can provide assistance when needed.

Adaptive Strategies:

Be flexible and willing to adapt your activities based on your current asthma status and environmental conditions. Have alternative exercises in mind for days when outdoor conditions are not ideal.

Asthma should not be a barrier to enjoying sports and physical activities. With careful planning, appropriate medical management, and a positive mindset, you can lead an active and fulfilling life. Embrace the benefits of exercise, listen to your body, and don't hesitate to seek support when needed.

CONCLUSION

Living with asthma can present its challenges, but it is entirely possible to lead a full, active, and vibrant life. This book has aimed to equip you with the knowledge and tools needed to manage your asthma effectively, enabling you to pursue your passions, achieve your goals, and enjoy your daily activities without being hindered by your condition.

Understanding Asthma

By comprehending the nature of asthma, its types, and how it affects your body, you gain the foundational knowledge necessary for effective management. Recognizing symptoms and triggers allows you to anticipate and prevent asthma attacks, ensuring that you remain in control of your health.

Partnering with Your Healthcare Team

Collaborating closely with your healthcare providers is crucial. They are your partners in managing asthma, offering invaluable insights, diagnostic tools, and personalized treatment plans. Your adherence to prescribed medications and techniques can significantly improve your quality of life, reducing the frequency and severity of asthma symptoms.

Building a Healthy Lifestyle

Incorporating healthy habits into your lifestyle is a powerful way to manage asthma. Identifying and avoiding triggers, both indoors and outdoors, helps create a safer environment. Embracing proper breathing techniques and relaxation strategies reduces stress and anxiety, which can exacerbate asthma symptoms. Furthermore, understanding the link between diet and asthma enables you to make informed food choices that support your respiratory health.

Staying Active

Physical activity is not only possible but beneficial for individuals with asthma. By choosing suitable activities, preparing adequately, and managing symptoms during exercise, you can enjoy the numerous advantages of an active lifestyle. Regular exercise enhances lung function, boosts the immune system, and improves overall fitness, contributing to better asthma control.

Mental and Emotional Wellbeing

Asthma can impact mental health, and vice versa. Managing stress, anxiety, and depression through relaxation techniques and building resilience fosters a positive outlook. Advocating for yourself in different settings, whether at school, work, or during travel, ensures that your needs are met, and you can participate fully in life's opportunities.

The Future of Asthma Management

The landscape of asthma management is continually evolving with emerging therapies and advancements. Staying informed about the latest research and developments allows you to benefit from new treatments and strategies. Reliable resources, support groups, and online communities provide a wealth of information and a sense of solidarity with others who understand your journey.

Celebrating Your Successes

Embrace a positive and empowering mindset. Celebrate your successes, no matter how small, and recognize your strength in overcoming challenges. Share your story to inspire others and contribute to a broader understanding of living well with asthma.

Final Thoughts

Asthma may be a part of your life, but it does not define you. With the right knowledge, support, and mindset, you can navigate its challenges and lead a fulfilling, breathtaking life. Remember, managing asthma is a continuous journey, but it is one you do not have to walk alone. Stay proactive, stay informed, and stay positive. Here's to your health and happiness as you embrace life with asthma!

GLOSSARY

1. Allergens: Substances that can cause an allergic reaction and trigger asthma symptoms, such as pollen, dust mites, mold, and pet dander.

2. Asthma Action Plan: A personalized plan developed with your healthcare provider to manage asthma, detailing medication use, trigger avoidance, and steps to take during an asthma attack.

3. Bronchodilators: Medications that relax the muscles around the airways, making it easier to breathe. These can be short-acting (for quick relief) or long-acting (for ongoing control).

4. Dust Mites: Microscopic organisms that live in household dust and can trigger asthma symptoms.

5. Inhaler: A device used to deliver asthma medication directly to the lungs. Common types include metered-dose inhalers (MDIs) and dry powder inhalers (DPIs).

7.   Inhaled   Corticosteroids: Anti-inflammatory medications that reduce swelling and mucus production in the airways, helping to prevent asthma symptoms.

8. Long-term Control Medications: Medications taken daily to manage and prevent asthma symptoms. These include inhaled corticosteroids, long-acting bronchodilators, and leukotriene modifiers.

9. Peak Flow Meter: A handheld device used to measure how well air moves out of your lungs, helping to monitor asthma control and detect early signs of an asthma attack.

10. Pollen: Fine particles released by plants that can trigger allergic reactions and asthma symptoms.

11. Rescue Medications: Fast-acting medications used to relieve acute asthma symptoms during an asthma attack. Commonly include short-acting bronchodilators.

12. Spirometry: A common test used to diagnose and monitor asthma, measuring how much air you can inhale and exhale, and how quickly you can exhale.

13. Triggers: Factors that can cause asthma symptoms or attacks, including allergens, irritants, respiratory infections, physical activity, and weather changes.

14. Weather Changes: Variations in temperature, humidity, and air quality that can exacerbate asthma symptoms.

15, Leukotriene Modifiers: Medications that block the action of leukotrienes, substances in the body that cause inflammation and constrict airways, helping to control asthma symptoms.

16. Nebulizer: A device that turns liquid asthma medication into a fine mist, which can be inhaled through a mask or mouthpiece.

17. Personalized Treatment Plan: A tailored approach to managing asthma, including specific medications, lifestyle adjustments, and strategies to avoid triggers, developed in collaboration with healthcare providers.

18. Symptom Tracking: The practice of recording asthma symptoms and their frequency to monitor asthma control and identify patterns or triggers.

19. Diaphragmatic Breathing: A breathing technique that involves deep, even breaths using the diaphragm, helping to strengthen the lungs and improve oxygen intake.

20. Pursed-Lip Breathing: A breathing technique that involves inhaling slowly through the nose and exhaling through pursed lips, helping to maintain open airways and reduce shortness of breath.

"Thanks for reading! If you enjoyed this book or found it useful, I'd be very grateful if you'd post a short review on Amazon. Your support really does make a difference and I read all the reviews personally so I can get your feedback and make this book even better.